CANCER

A Doctor's Practical Guide to Prevention & Early Detection

Dr Prabhat Das

MD, PhD, FACP

Better Health with Dr Das Series

Hardcover ISBN: 978-1-971672-67-0

Paperback ISBN: 978-1-971672-66-3

eBook ISBN: 978-1-971672-65-6

Printed in the United States of America

Disclaimer

This book is intended solely for educational and informational purposes. It is not meant to replace personal medical advice, diagnosis, or treatment.

Although I am a licensed physician, reading this book does not establish a doctor-patient relationship. Each individual's health condition, medical history, and risk factors are unique. Any medical decision should be made in partnership with your own healthcare professional who understands your specific situation.

Medical science is continually advancing. New research and updated guidelines may lead to changes in recommendations over time.

TABLE OF CONTENTS:

About the Author

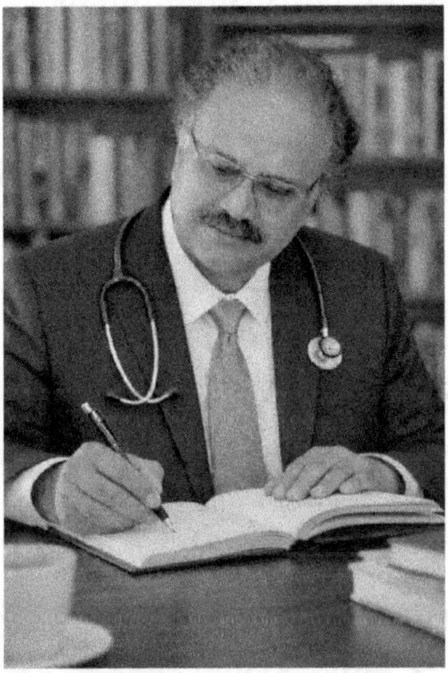

I am Dr Prabhat Das, MD, PhD, FACP. My journey in medicine began in India and, over the past thirty-five years, has continued in the United States, where I have had the privilege of caring for patients across a wide range of medical settings. I am trained in Internal Medicine, Pulmonary Diseases, and Critical Care. For me, medicine has never been just a profession. It has been a lifelong commitment shaped by learning, service, and a deep respect for the trust patients place in their physician.

Over the years, I have had the honor of caring for patients in many different situations. I have seen individuals in my office for routine concerns, treated urgent conditions in busy emergency rooms, managed serious illnesses in the hospital, and cared for critically ill patients in intensive care units. Each setting has taught me something valuable. Each patient has added to my understanding of what it truly means to care for another human being.

But one lesson has stood above all others. Medicine is not only about tests, diagnoses, or treatments. It is about people. It is about listening carefully, understanding fears that are often left unspoken, and guiding patients through uncertainty with clarity and compassion. Again and again, I have seen that what people want most is simple, trustworthy information. They want to understand what is happening in their bodies. They want to feel confident about the decisions they are making for their health and for their families.

These experiences have deeply shaped how I think about health, illness, prevention, and the human side of healing.

That is the reason behind the '**Better Health with Dr Das Series'.** Through these books, I hope to reach individuals I may never meet in person but who are searching for clear and reliable guidance. In today's world, health information is everywhere, yet much of it is confusing, overwhelming, and sometimes misleading. My goal is to cut through that noise and present important medical topics in a way that is simple, practical, and reassuring.

Every page of this series is guided by two foundations: reliable scientific knowledge and decades of real-world clinical experience. I want you, the reader, to feel informed, confident, and empowered. Not overwhelmed. Not confused. But clear about what you can do, step by step, to improve your health.

If even one reader feels less anxious, more informed, or better prepared to take control of their health after reading these books, then this work has served its purpose.

Helping people live healthier, longer, more confident and better-informed lives remains one of the greatest privileges of my life.

INTRODUCTION: Understanding Cancer Without Fear

A Word That Changes Everything

There are certain moments in life that quietly divide time into "before" and "after."

For many people, hearing the word **cancer** is one of those moments.

I have seen this countless times in my years of medical practice. A patient walks into the room with a concern. We talk. We examine. We review tests. And then, when the possibility of cancer is mentioned, something shifts.

The room becomes silent.

Eyes search for answers.

Fear appears, even before the facts are fully known.

This reaction is deeply human. It comes from what we have seen, what we have heard, and what we imagine cancer to be.

But over the years, I have also witnessed something equally powerful.

I have seen that fear change.

I have seen patients move from confusion to clarity. From helplessness to control. From anxiety to informed decision-making.

And almost always, that change begins with one thing.

Understanding.

Why This Book Is Important

In today's world, information is everywhere.

You can search online and find thousands of articles, opinions, videos, and personal stories about cancer. Some of this information is useful. Much of it is incomplete, outdated, or simply incorrect.

This creates a problem.

Instead of clarity, people feel overwhelmed. Instead of confidence, they feel uncertain.

Some delay medical care because they are afraid.
Some believe myths that are not supported by science.
Some lose valuable time searching for answers in the wrong places.

As a physician who has spent decades caring for patients in clinics, hospitals, and intensive care units, I have seen the consequences of this confusion.

That is why I felt the need to write this book.

What This Book Will Do for You

This book is written with a simple goal.

To help you understand cancer in a clear, practical, and honest way.

By the time you finish reading, you will have a solid understanding of:

- What cancer really is
- Why it develops
- What increases your risk
- What you can do to reduce that risk
- How to recognize early warning signs
- The role of screening and early detection
- What happens after a diagnosis
- The different treatment options
- How to live during and after treatment

More importantly, you will feel more prepared.

You will know what to do, and just as importantly, what not to do.

How This Book Is Different

This is not a textbook.

You will not find unnecessary medical jargon or complicated explanations that are difficult to follow.

Instead, I have written this as I would speak to a patient sitting in front of me.

Simple. Clear. Honest.

Whenever medical terms are needed, they are explained in a way that makes sense. Each chapter builds on the previous one, so that you gradually develop a complete understanding.

I have also taken great care to ensure that all information in this book is based on reliable medical knowledge and current understanding from established sources such as major cancer research organizations and clinical guidelines.

At the same time, I have written this in a way that feels human.

Because cancer is not just a medical condition. It is a personal experience.

A Balanced Approach: Neither Fear Nor False Hope

There are two extremes that I often see.

One is fear.

The belief that cancer always leads to suffering and death.

The other is false reassurance.

The idea that cancer can be easily cured by simple remedies or that it is not serious.

Both are incorrect.

Cancer is a serious condition. It deserves attention, respect, and timely action.

But it is also a condition where:

- Many cases can be prevented
- Many can be detected early
- Many can be treated effectively

The correct approach lies in understanding, not extremes.

What I Want You to Remember from the Beginning

If you remember only a few things from this book, let them be these:

- Not all cancers are the same
- Early detection can change outcomes
- Lifestyle choices matter
- Reliable information is essential
- You are not helpless

These are simple ideas, but they are powerful.

A Personal Note to You

As you read this book, I want you to feel that you are not alone.

Think of this as a conversation between us.

If you were sitting in my office, I would explain these concepts to you step by step. I would answer your questions. I would guide you without creating unnecessary fear.

That is exactly what I have tried to do here.

Take your time with this book.

Read it slowly. Reflect on it. Share it with your family if you wish.

Understanding cancer does not eliminate all uncertainty. But it replaces confusion with clarity.

And that is the first and most important step.

What Comes Next

In the next chapter, we will begin with the most basic and important question:

What exactly is cancer?

We will break it down in a simple way, so that you can clearly understand how it begins and how it behaves.

Once you understand that, everything else will become easier.

Let us begin this journey with clarity, not fear.

CHAPTER 1: Cancer: Understanding the Fear and Finding Clarity

Why This Word Feels So Heavy

There are few words in medicine that carry as much emotional weight as the word **cancer**.

In my years of practice, I have seen how this single word can change the atmosphere in a room within seconds. A conversation that was calm becomes tense. Faces become serious. Questions appear, even if they are not immediately spoken.

"Is this serious?"
"Will I survive?"
"What should I do now?"

This reaction is natural. It does not come from weakness. It comes from what we have seen, heard, and experienced over time.

Many people associate cancer with suffering, uncertainty, and loss. These impressions are often shaped by past experiences, sometimes from many years ago, when treatment options were limited.

But medicine has changed.

And understanding this change is the first step toward reducing fear.

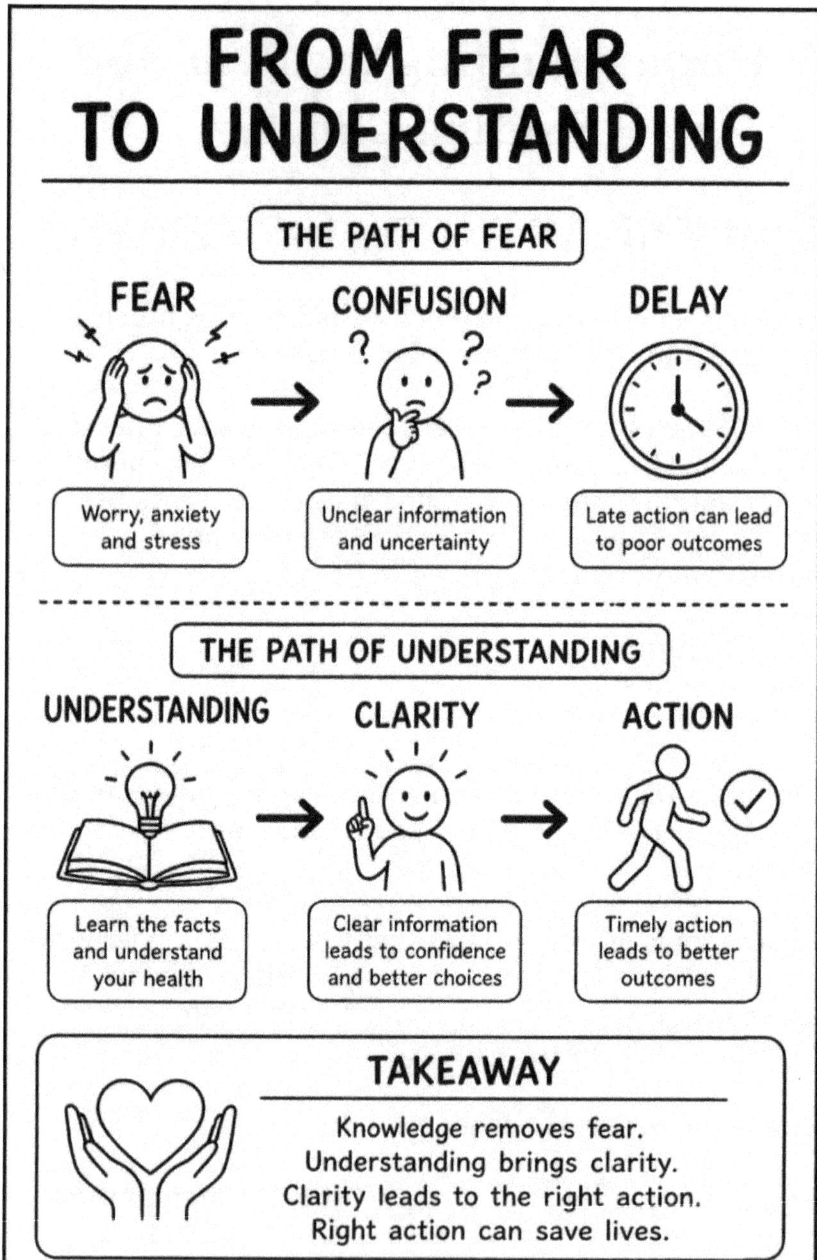
FROM FEAR TO UNDERSTANDING
THE PATH OF FEAR
FEAR
Worry, anxiety and stress
CONFUSION
Unclear information and uncertainty
DELAY
Late action can lead to poor outcomes
THE PATH OF UNDERSTANDING
UNDERSTANDING
Learn the facts and understand your health
CLARITY
Clear information leads to confidence and better choices
ACTION
Timely action leads to better outcomes
TAKEAWAY
Knowledge removes fear.
Understanding brings clarity.
Clarity leads to the right action.
Right action can save lives.

Fear Often Comes from Not Knowing

When something is not clearly understood, it often appears larger and more frightening than it actually is.

Cancer is a perfect example of this.

People hear different opinions from different sources. A friend shares a story. The internet provides endless information, much of it incomplete or misleading. Old beliefs continue to circulate even when they are no longer true.

This creates confusion.

Some people assume that cancer always leads to death.
Some believe in unproven treatments.
Some ignore symptoms because they are afraid to face the possibility.

In all these situations, the real problem is not just the disease.

It is the lack of clear understanding.

Cancer Today: A Different Reality

It is important to pause and recognize how much cancer care has improved.

There was a time when many cancers were detected late and treatment options were limited. Outcomes were often poor.

Today, the situation is very different.

- Many cancers can be detected early through screening
- Treatments are more precise and targeted
- Side effects are better managed
- Survival rates have improved in many cancers

I have personally cared for patients who were diagnosed with cancer and continued to live full and meaningful lives. Some returned to their normal routines. Others adapted and moved forward with strength and dignity.

This does not mean cancer is no longer serious.

It means that cancer is no longer what it used to be.

Understanding Reduces Fear

Let me share something I have observed repeatedly.

When patients first hear about cancer, fear is often high.

But when they begin to understand:

- What type of cancer it is

- What stage it is
- What treatment options are available

something changes.

The fear begins to settle.

Clarity replaces confusion.

Patients begin to ask better questions. They participate in decisions. They move forward with more confidence.

Understanding does not remove the seriousness of cancer.

But it gives you control.

A Practical Example

Consider two individuals.

One notices a symptom but ignores it because of fear. Months pass. The condition progresses.

Another notices the same symptom but seeks medical advice early. The problem is identified sooner, and treatment is simpler.

The disease may be similar.

The outcome is very different.

The difference lies in awareness and action.

What This Book Will Help You Do

This book is written to guide you step by step.

By the time you finish, you will:

- Understand what cancer is in simple terms
- Know why it develops
- Recognize risk factors
- Learn how to reduce your risk
- Understand early warning signs
- Know when and how to get screened
- Understand diagnosis and treatment
- Learn how to live during and after treatment

Most importantly, you will feel more prepared.

Doctor's Pearl

Understanding cancer is the first step toward reducing fear and taking control.

Myth vs Fact

Myth: Cancer always means death.
Fact: Many cancers are treatable, and some are curable, especially when detected early.

Common Mistake to Avoid

Ignoring symptoms or delaying medical evaluation because of fear.

Red Flag Warning

Any persistent, unexplained change in your body should be evaluated without delay.

Key Points

- The fear of cancer is often greater than the reality
- Lack of understanding increases anxiety
- Cancer care has improved significantly
- Early detection can change outcomes
- Awareness leads to better decisions

Chapter Summary

Cancer is one of the most feared medical conditions, largely because of uncertainty and misunderstanding. While it remains a serious disease, advances in modern medicine have significantly improved detection and treatment.

Understanding the condition allows you to move from fear to clarity and from confusion to informed action.

Action Plan

- Do not panic when you hear about cancer
- Seek reliable and accurate information
- Pay attention to your body
- Do not delay medical consultation
- Maintain a balanced and practical approach

Bridge to Next Chapter

Now that we have addressed the fear and confusion surrounding cancer, the next step is to understand the condition itself.

In the next chapter, we will clearly explain what cancer is and how it begins, in a simple and easy-to-understand way.

CHAPTER 2: What Cancer Really Is: A Simple and Clear Explanation

Start with the Basics: Your Body's Cells

To understand cancer, we must begin with something simple.

Your body is made up of trillions of cells. These cells are constantly working, growing, dividing, and replacing themselves.

It is a beautifully organized system.

- Cells grow only when needed
- They divide in a controlled way
- Old or damaged cells die and are replaced

This balance keeps your body healthy.

Most of the time, this system works perfectly.

Cancer begins when this balance is lost.

When Cells Stop Following the Rules

A cancer cell is not something foreign.

It is a normal cell that has changed.

Instead of following the body's instructions, it begins to behave differently.

- It grows when it should not
- It divides without control
- It does not die when it is supposed to

Over time, these abnormal cells accumulate.

At first, this process is silent. You feel nothing. But gradually, it can lead to the formation of a mass, which we call a tumor.

This process usually takes years, sometimes decades.

The Role of DNA: The Cell's Instruction Manual

Inside every cell is DNA.

You can think of DNA as the instruction manual that tells the cell what to do.

Sometimes, this DNA becomes damaged.

In most cases, the body repairs this damage. But occasionally, the repair is not perfect.

If the damage affects important parts of the DNA that control growth, the cell begins to grow abnormally.

Over time, these abnormal cells multiply and form cancer.

This is the basic mechanism behind most cancers.

Not Every Growth Is Cancer

This is an important point that reduces unnecessary fear.

Not every lump or growth is cancer.

There are two main types of growths:

Benign Tumors

- Non-cancerous
- Grow slowly
- Do not spread

Malignant Tumors (Cancer)

- Grow more aggressively
- Can invade nearby tissues
- Can spread to other parts of the body

Understanding this difference helps you approach symptoms more calmly and wisely.

What Cancer Really Is

Cancer begins when normal cells grow and divide in an uncontrolled way.

NORMAL CELL

Cells grow, divide and die in a controlled way.

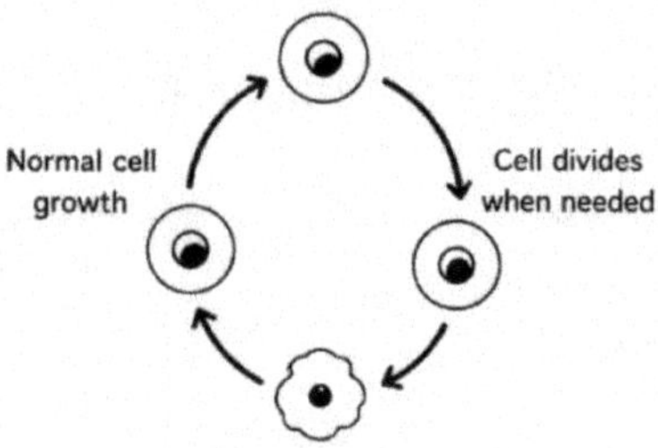

Old or damaged cells die and are removed

Result: Healthy tissue works normally.

CANCER CELL

Cells grow and divide without control.

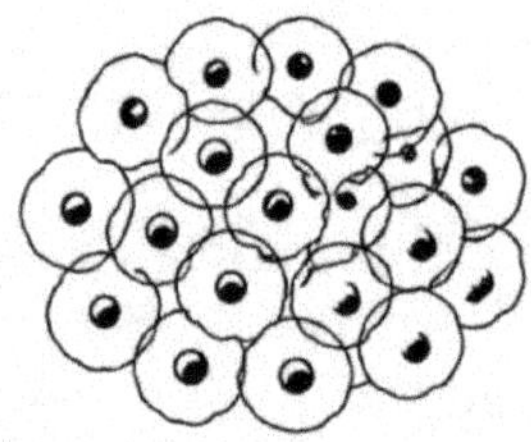

Abnormal cells continue to divide. Old or damaged cells do not die. They form a mass called a tumor.

Result: Tumor can grow, damage normal tissue and spread.

HOW CANCER CAN SPREAD

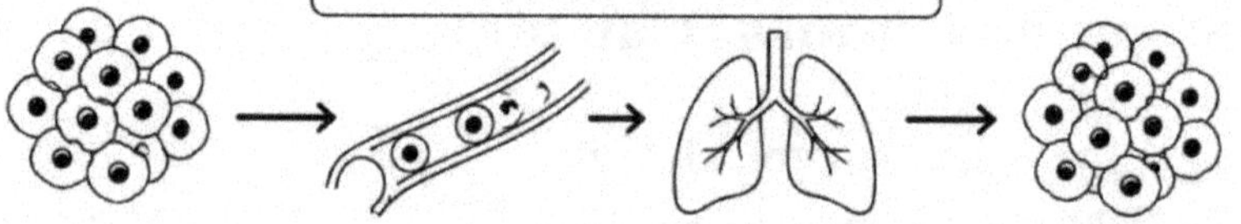

Tumor in original organ → Cancer cells enter the blood or lymph vessels → Cancer cells travel to other parts of the body → New tumors may form in other organs (metastasis)

KEY POINTS

- Cancer is not one disease, but many different diseases.
- It starts when normal cells change and grow out of control.
- Early detection and proper treatment can save lives.

How Cancer Spreads: Understanding Metastasis

One of the defining features of cancer is its ability to spread.

At first, cancer usually begins in one location.

Over time, some cancer cells can break away and travel through the bloodstream or the lymphatic system. They can then settle in other organs and form new tumors.

This process is called metastasis.

For example, a cancer that starts in the lung may spread to the brain or bones.

Once cancer spreads, treatment becomes more complex.

That is why early detection is so important.

Cancer Is Not One Disease

Another important point to understand is this.

Cancer is not a single disease.

It is a group of many different diseases.

Some common categories include:

- **Carcinomas**: cancers of organs such as breast, lung, and colon
- **Sarcomas**: cancers of bone and muscle
- **Leukemias**: cancers of the blood
- **Lymphomas**: cancers of the immune system

Each type behaves differently. Each responds differently to treatment.

This is why treatment is always individualized.

Why Some Cancers Behave Differently

Not all cancers grow at the same rate.

Some grow slowly and may remain stable for years.

Others grow rapidly and require urgent treatment.

This depends on:

- The type of cancer
- Genetic changes in the cells
- The body's response

This explains why two people with cancer can have very different experiences.

A Practical Example

Consider two individuals.

One develops a slow-growing prostate cancer that remains limited for many years.

Another develops a more aggressive cancer that spreads quickly.

Both are cancers.

But their behavior, treatment, and outcomes are very different.

Understanding this helps avoid unnecessary fear and generalization.

Doctor's Pearl

Cancer begins as a small change in a single cell, but early detection can prevent it from becoming a serious problem.

Myth vs Fact

Myth: Every tumor is cancer.
Fact: Many tumors are benign and not harmful.

Common Mistake to Avoid

Ignoring a new lump or body change without proper evaluation.

Red Flag Warning

Any new, growing, or persistent lump should be evaluated by a doctor.

Key Points

- Cancer begins with abnormal cell growth
- It develops due to changes in DNA
- Not all growths are cancer
- Cancer can spread to other parts of the body
- Different cancers behave differently

Chapter Summary

Cancer develops when normal cells lose control and begin to grow and divide abnormally. This process is driven by changes in DNA and usually occurs over a long period.

Not all growths are cancer, and different cancers behave in different ways. Understanding these basics provides a strong foundation for everything that follows.

Action Plan

- Do not panic if you notice a lump, but do not ignore it
- Pay attention to changes in your body
- Seek medical advice for persistent symptoms
- Understand the importance of early detection
- Stay informed through reliable sources

Bridge to Next Chapter

Now that you understand what cancer is, the next question is:

Why does it happen?

In the next chapter, we will clearly explain the causes of cancer, including lifestyle, environment, and genetic factors, in a practical and understandable way.

CHAPTER 3: Why Cancer Happens: Understanding the Real Causes Without Blame

The Question Almost Everyone Asks

Soon after a diagnosis, one question comes up again and again.

"Why did this happen to me?"

It is a very human question. When something serious enters our life, we look for a reason. Many people go back through their habits, their diet, their past decisions.

Some feel guilty. Others feel confused, especially if they have lived a healthy life.

Let me say this clearly.

In most cases, cancer does not happen because of one single cause.

It develops slowly, over many years, due to a combination of factors.

Understanding this helps remove unnecessary guilt and allows you to focus on what truly matters.

At the Root: Changes in DNA Over Time

As we discussed earlier, cancer begins when there are changes in the DNA of a cell.

DNA controls how cells grow and behave.

These changes may occur due to:

- Natural aging
- Environmental exposures
- Lifestyle factors
- Certain infections

Most of the time, the body repairs these changes. But sometimes, small errors remain.

Over time, these errors can accumulate and lead to cancer.

This process usually takes years, often decades.

Aging: The Most Common Risk Factor

One of the most important factors is age.

As we grow older:

- Our cells divide repeatedly

- Small DNA changes accumulate
- The body's repair mechanisms become less efficient

This is why cancer is more common after the age of 50.

Aging is a natural process. It cannot be changed. But it explains why screening becomes more important as we get older.

Lifestyle Factors: Where You Have Control

A significant number of cancers are linked to lifestyle.

This is important, because it means risk can be reduced.

Tobacco

Tobacco is the most important preventable cause of cancer.

It is linked to cancers of the lung, mouth, throat, bladder, pancreas, and more.

Diet and Body Weight

A diet high in processed foods and low in fruits and vegetables can increase risk.

Excess body weight is associated with several cancers, including breast and colon cancer.

Physical Inactivity

Lack of regular activity contributes to weight gain and affects overall health.

Alcohol

Regular alcohol use increases the risk of cancers such as liver, breast, and esophageal cancer.

Small, consistent changes in these areas can have a meaningful impact.

Environmental Factors: Risks Around Us

We arc all exposed to environmental factors.

Some of these may increase cancer risk.

Examples include:

- Air pollution
- Ultraviolet radiation from the sun
- Certain workplace chemicals such as asbestos

You may not be able to control all exposures, but awareness helps you take precautions when possible.

How Cancer Develops Over Time

Cancer usually does not appear overnight.
It develops slowly over many years.

1 DNA DAMAGE

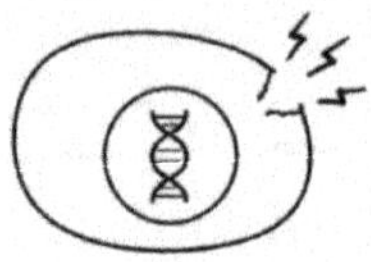

Our DNA can be damaged by tobacco, chemicals, radiation, infections, or other factors.

2 FAILED REPAIR

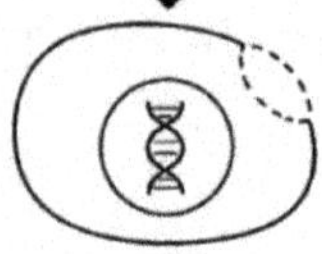

Normally, the cell repairs the damage. Sometimes the repair fails.

3 ABNORMAL CELLS

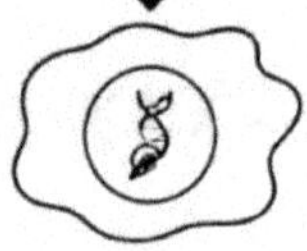

Damaged cells start growing and dividing in an uncontrolled way.

4 TUMOR FORMATION

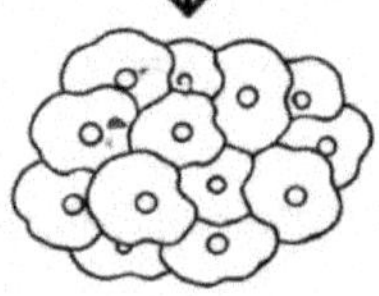

Abnormal cells form a mass called a tumor. It can grow and damage nearby tissues.

5 CANCER SPREAD

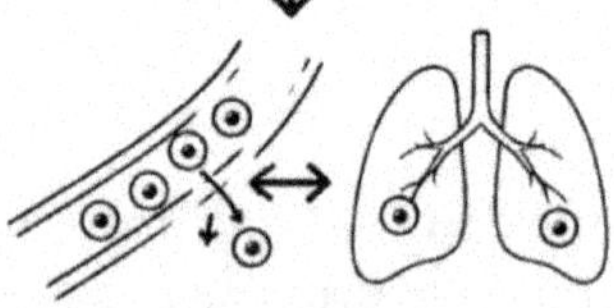

Cancer cells can break away, travel in blood or lymph, and form new tumors in other parts of the body.

KEY TAKEAWAY

Cancer develops in steps over many years.
Avoid risk factors. Get regular check-ups.
Early detection can stop cancer early.

Infections That Increase Cancer Risk

Some infections are known to increase cancer risk.

Human Papillomavirus (HPV)

Linked to cervical cancer and some throat cancers.

Hepatitis B and C

Associated with liver cancer.

Helicobacter pylori

Linked to stomach cancer.

The important point is that some of these risks can be reduced through vaccination and early treatment.

Genetics and Family History

Some people inherit genes that increase their risk.

If close family members have had cancer, especially at a younger age, your risk may be higher.

But it is important to remember:

- Most cancers are not inherited
- Having a family history does not mean cancer is certain

It simply means that awareness and early screening become more important.

When There Is No Clear Cause

In many cases, no single cause can be identified.

This can be frustrating.

But it reflects the complex nature of cancer.

Multiple small factors may combine over time, and not all of them are fully understood.

Blaming yourself is neither accurate nor helpful.

A Practical Example

One person has a long history of smoking and develops lung cancer.

Another has never smoked but still develops lung cancer.

The first situation has a clear risk factor.

The second may involve a combination of environmental exposure, genetic factors, and natural DNA changes.

Both are real.

This is why cancer cannot always be explained by a single reason.

Doctor's Pearl

Cancer usually develops due to a combination of factors over time, not a single cause.

Myth vs Fact

Myth: Cancer happens only because of unhealthy habits.
Fact: While lifestyle plays a major role, many factors, including age and genetics, contribute.

Common Mistake to Avoid

Blaming yourself instead of focusing on understanding and taking action.

Red Flag Warning

A strong family history of cancer should prompt discussion with your doctor and appropriate screening.

Key Points

- Cancer begins with changes in DNA
- Aging is a major risk factor
- Lifestyle factors play a significant role
- Environmental exposures contribute
- Some infections increase risk
- Not all cancers have a clear cause

Chapter Summary

Cancer develops due to a combination of factors that lead to changes in DNA over time. These factors include aging, lifestyle, environmental exposures, infections, and genetics.

Understanding these causes helps reduce unnecessary guilt and allows you to focus on prevention and early detection.

Action Plan

- Avoid tobacco completely
- Maintain a healthy weight
- Eat a balanced diet
- Stay physically active
- Limit alcohol intake
- Stay updated on vaccinations
- Be aware of your family history
- Follow screening recommendations

Bridge to Next Chapter

Now that you understand why cancer happens, the next important step is to understand risk in a practical way.

In the next chapter, we will discuss cancer risk factors and what you can and cannot change.

CHAPTER 4: Cancer Risk Factors: What You Can Change and What You Cannot

Understanding Risk Without Anxiety

After learning why cancer happens, most people begin to wonder:

"What is my risk?"

This is an important question. But it must be approached in the right way.

Risk does not mean certainty.

Having a risk factor does not mean you will develop cancer. At the same time, having no obvious risk does not guarantee that cancer cannot occur.

The purpose of understanding risk is not to create fear. It is to guide your actions.

Two Types of Risk Factors

All cancer risk factors can be broadly divided into two groups.

Modifiable Risk Factors

These are factors you can change.

Non-Modifiable Risk Factors

These are factors you cannot change.

This distinction is very important.

You should not worry about what you cannot change. Focus your attention on what you can improve.

Tobacco: The Most Important Preventable Risk

If there is one factor that clearly stands out, it is tobacco.

Tobacco use is strongly linked to many cancers, including:

- Lung
- Mouth
- Throat
- Bladder
- Pancreas

Even secondhand smoke increases risk.

The positive message is this:

Stopping tobacco reduces risk, even after years of use.

It is never too late to quit.

Alcohol: A Common but Overlooked Risk

Alcohol is often seen as a normal part of social life.

However, regular use increases the risk of several cancers, including:

- Liver
- Breast
- Esophagus

The risk increases with the amount consumed.

Moderation is important.

Body Weight, Diet, and Physical Activity

These three factors are closely connected.

Excess Body Weight

Being overweight increases the risk of several cancers, including breast and colon cancer.

Diet

A diet high in processed foods and low in fruits and vegetables can increase risk.

Physical Inactivity

Lack of activity contributes to weight gain and reduces overall health.

A Practical Approach

- Eat balanced meals
- Limit processed foods
- Stay physically active

You do not need perfection. You need consistency.

Sun Exposure and Skin Cancer

Excessive exposure to sunlight, especially ultraviolet radiation, increases the risk of skin cancer.

Simple precautions can reduce this risk:

- Avoid prolonged exposure during peak sunlight hours
- Use sunscreen
- Wear protective clothing

These habits are simple but effective.

Cancer Risk Factors

Some risk factors can be changed.
Some cannot.

WHAT YOU CAN CHANGE

- Tobacco use
- Alcohol use
- Unhealthy diet
- Excess body weight
- Physical inactivity

WHAT YOU CANNOT CHANGE

- Increasing age
- Family history of cancer
- Genetic factors
- Gender

TAKEAWAY

Focus on what you can change.
Small daily actions reduce risk.

Environmental and Workplace Risks

Some risks come from the environment.

Examples include:

- Air pollution
- Industrial chemicals
- Asbestos exposure

You may not have complete control over these factors, but awareness allows you to take precautions where possible.

Infections and Cancer Risk

Certain infections are linked to cancer.

Examples include:

- HPV, associated with cervical and throat cancers
- Hepatitis B and C, associated with liver cancer

Vaccination and early treatment can reduce these risks.

Family History and Genetics

Some people have a higher risk due to inherited genes.

If close family members have had cancer, especially at a younger age, your risk may be higher.

However:

- Most cancers are not inherited
- A family history does not mean cancer is certain

It simply means that you should be more aware and follow appropriate screening.

Age and Gender

Certain risk factors cannot be changed.

Age

Cancer risk increases as we grow older.

Gender

Some cancers are more common in men, others in women.

These factors help guide screening and prevention.

Balancing Control and Acceptance

A healthy approach to risk includes both action and acceptance.

- Act on what you can change
- Accept what you cannot

This balanced approach reduces unnecessary anxiety.

A Practical Example

Two individuals have similar family histories.

One ignores lifestyle factors.

The other improves diet, activity, and overall health.

Even with the same genetic background, their risk and outcomes may differ.

Doctor's Pearl

You cannot control every risk, but you can control the most important ones.

Myth vs Fact

Myth: If cancer runs in the family, nothing can be done.
Fact: Lifestyle changes and early screening can significantly reduce risk.

Common Mistake to Avoid

Focusing only on genetic risk while ignoring lifestyle factors.

Red Flag Warning

A strong family history of cancer should be discussed with your doctor.

Key Points

- Risk does not mean certainty
- Some risk factors can be changed
- Tobacco is the most important avoidable risk
- Diet, weight, and activity matter
- Environmental and genetic factors contribute
- Awareness leads to better prevention

Chapter Summary

Cancer risk is influenced by a combination of factors. Some can be changed, such as lifestyle habits, while others, such as age and genetics, cannot.

Understanding risk allows you to take practical steps to reduce your chances of developing cancer.

Action Plan

- Avoid tobacco completely
- Limit alcohol intake
- Maintain a healthy weight
- Eat a balanced diet
- Stay physically active
- Protect your skin from excessive sun exposure
- Be aware of your family history
- Follow screening recommendations

Bridge to Next Chapter

Now that you understand cancer risk, the next step is to focus on prevention.

In the next chapter, we will discuss practical steps you can take to reduce your risk and protect your health over time.

CHAPTER 5: Can Cancer Be Prevented? Practical Steps That Truly Work

A Question Patients Ask Me Often

One of the most common questions I hear is simple and direct:

"Doctor, can cancer really be prevented?"

The honest answer is balanced.

Not all cancers can be prevented. But many can be.

That distinction is very important.

Prevention is not about guarantees. It is about reducing risk in a meaningful and practical way.

When you understand this, prevention becomes empowering rather than overwhelming.

The Most Powerful Step: Stay Away from Tobacco

If I had to choose one single action that makes the greatest difference, it would be this.

Avoid tobacco completely.

Tobacco use is linked to multiple cancers, including:

- Lung
- Mouth
- Throat
- Bladder
- Pancreas

Even exposure to secondhand smoke increases risk.

The encouraging part is this.

Stopping tobacco use at any stage reduces risk. The earlier you stop, the greater the benefit.

This is one of the most important decisions you can make for your long-term health.

Healthy Eating: Keep It Realistic and Sustainable

There is no single "anti-cancer diet."

But there are clear patterns that support better health.

Focus on:

- Fresh fruits and vegetables
- Whole grains
- Moderate portion sizes

- Limiting processed and red meat

Avoid extreme diets that are difficult to maintain.

Simple, consistent habits are far more effective.

Maintain a Healthy Body Weight

Excess body weight is linked to several cancers, including breast, colon, and uterine cancer.

Weight control is not about short-term dieting.

It is about long-term habits.

Even small, steady improvements in eating and activity can make a meaningful difference.

Stay Physically Active

Physical activity plays a key role in prevention.

It helps:

- Maintain weight
- Improve overall body function
- Support the immune system

You do not need intense exercise.

Regular movement such as walking, stretching, or light activity is enough to provide benefit.

Consistency matters more than intensity.

Limit Alcohol Intake

Alcohol is associated with an increased risk of several cancers.

The risk rises with higher consumption.

If you drink, do so in moderation. If you do not drink, there is no need to start.

Vaccination: A Powerful Preventive Tool

Some cancers can be prevented through vaccination.

HPV Vaccine

Protects against human papillomavirus, which is linked to cervical cancer and certain throat cancers.

Hepatitis B Vaccine

Reduces the risk of liver cancer by preventing chronic infection.

These are safe, effective, and important preventive measures.

Protect Your Skin

Skin cancer is one of the most preventable cancers.

Simple steps include:

- Avoiding excessive sun exposure
- Using sunscreen
- Wearing protective clothing

These habits are easy to adopt and highly effective.

Avoid False Promises and "Miracle" Claims

You may come across claims about special foods, supplements, or treatments that promise to prevent cancer.

Be cautious.

There is no single food or supplement that can guarantee prevention.

Reliable prevention comes from consistent, evidence-based habits.

Cancer Prevention

Healthy choices today can help prevent cancer tomorrow.

1 DO NOT USE TOBACCO

Avoid all forms of tobacco.

2 EAT A HEALTHY DIET

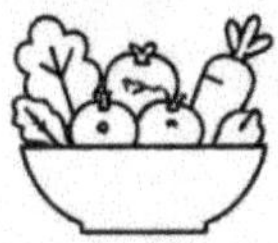

Eat more fruits, vegetables, whole grains and beans.

3 BE PHYSICALLY ACTIVE

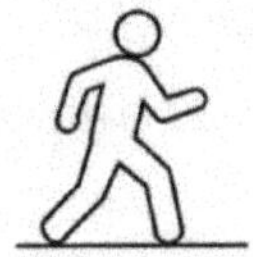

Be active every day. Limit sitting time.

4 MAINTAIN A HEALTHY WEIGHT

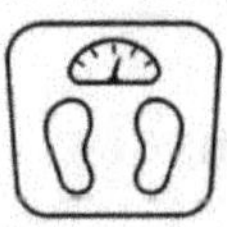

Keep your weight in a healthy range.

5 LIMIT ALCOHOL

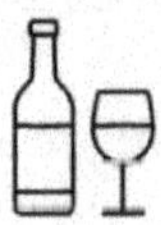

If you drink, limit your alcohol intake.

6 PROTECT YOURSELF FROM THE SUN

Use shade, clothing and sunscreen.

7 GET VACCINATED

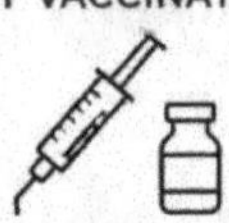

Hepatitis B and HPV vaccines can help prevent cancer.

8 GET REGULAR CHECK-UPS

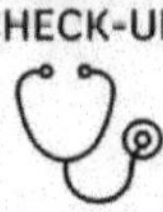

Screening can find cancer early when it is easier to treat.

9 AVOID HARMFUL SUBSTANCES

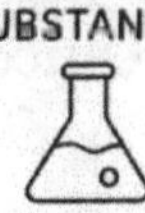

Avoid exposure to harmful chemicals and radiation when possible.

KEY TAKEAWAY

You have the power to reduce your risk. Small healthy choices can make a big difference.

Prevention Is a Way of Life

Prevention is not something you do for a few weeks.

It is a long-term approach to living.

Small, steady changes over time have the greatest impact.

You do not need perfection.

You need consistency.

A Practical Example

Two individuals live very different lifestyles.

One continues unhealthy habits without change.

Another makes gradual improvements in diet, activity, and daily routine.

Over time, these small differences can significantly influence cancer risk.

Doctor's Pearl

Prevention is built on simple, consistent habits, not extreme changes.

Myth vs Fact

Myth: A single food or supplement can prevent cancer.
Fact: Prevention depends on overall lifestyle, not one factor.

Common Mistake to Avoid

Looking for quick solutions instead of building long-term healthy habits.

Red Flag Warning

Avoid relying on unproven methods or "miracle cures" for prevention.

Key Points

- Many cancers can be prevented
- Avoiding tobacco is the most important step
- Healthy diet and weight matter
- Physical activity supports prevention
- Alcohol should be limited
- Vaccination can prevent certain cancers
- Consistency is key

Chapter Summary

Cancer prevention is not absolute, but it is powerful. By making informed lifestyle choices, you can significantly reduce your risk.

Avoiding tobacco, maintaining a healthy weight, staying active, eating a balanced diet, limiting alcohol, protecting your skin, and following vaccination recommendations are key strategies.

Action Plan

- Avoid tobacco completely
- Eat a balanced, natural diet
- Maintain a healthy weight
- Stay physically active
- Limit alcohol intake
- Follow vaccination guidelines
- Protect your skin from excessive sun exposure
- Avoid unproven health claims

Bridge to Next Chapter

Even with the best preventive efforts, it is important to recognize early warning signs.

In the next chapter, we will discuss symptoms that should never be ignored and when to seek medical attention.

CHAPTER 6: Early Warning Signs You Should Never Ignore

Your Body Often Speaks Quietly First

One of the most important lessons I have learned over the years is simple.

The body usually gives early signals before a serious problem develops.

These signals are often subtle. They may not cause pain. They may come and go. Because of this, they are easy to ignore.

Many patients later tell me, "I noticed it, but I thought it was nothing."
Others say, "I did not want to worry about it."

This is where delay begins.

Paying attention to early warning signs does not mean living in fear. It means staying aware.

The Golden Rule: Persistence Matters

Almost every symptom we discuss in this chapter can occur in common, non-cancer conditions.

That is why the symptom alone is not the most important factor.

The pattern is.

You should pay attention when a symptom is:

- Persistent
- Unexplained
- Gradually worsening

This simple rule helps you stay alert without unnecessary anxiety.

Unexplained Weight Loss and Persistent Fatigue

Losing weight without trying may seem positive at first, but it should be taken seriously if there is no clear reason.

Persistent fatigue is another important signal.

This is not normal tiredness. It is a sense of exhaustion that does not improve with rest.

These symptoms are not specific to cancer, but when they continue, they require evaluation.

Lumps, Swelling, and Visible Changes

A new lump is one of the most noticeable warning signs.

Common examples include:

- A lump in the breast
- Swelling in the neck
- A mass in the abdomen

Most lumps are not cancer, but every new or changing lump should be checked.

Also watch for:

- Skin changes
- Non-healing sores
- Changes in moles

Visible changes are often easier to detect, but they are sometimes ignored.

Persistent Cough, Hoarseness, or Difficulty Swallowing

Symptoms related to the lungs and throat deserve attention when they persist.

Watch for:

- A cough that does not go away
- Hoarseness lasting more than a few weeks
- Difficulty swallowing

These symptoms are often caused by common conditions, but persistence is the key concern.

Changes in Bowel or Bladder Habits

Your daily habits can provide important clues.

Be alert to:

- Persistent constipation or diarrhea
- Blood in stool or urine
- Change in stool size or shape
- Increased or difficult urination

Even small changes can be important if they continue.

Unusual Bleeding or Discharge

Bleeding without a clear reason should always be evaluated.

Examples include:

- Blood in sputum
- Blood in stool

- Vaginal bleeding after menopause
- Unusual discharge

These are important warning signs.

Pain That Does Not Go Away

Pain is often thought of as a late symptom, but it can sometimes appear earlier.

Persistent pain that:

- Has no clear cause
- Gradually worsens
- Interferes with daily life

should not be ignored.

Pain is the body's signal that something needs attention.

Silent Cancers: When There Are No Symptoms

It is important to understand that not all cancers produce early symptoms.

Some cancers remain silent for a long time.

This is why screening is so important.

Relying only on symptoms is not enough.

When Should You See a Doctor?

A simple and practical rule can guide you.

If a symptom:

- Lasts more than a few weeks
- Has no clear explanation
- Is getting worse

you should seek medical advice.

Early consultation is a sign of awareness, not fear.

A Practical Example

One person notices blood in the stool but ignores it.

Another notices the same symptom and seeks medical advice early.

The second person has a much better chance of early detection and effective treatment.

The difference is timing.

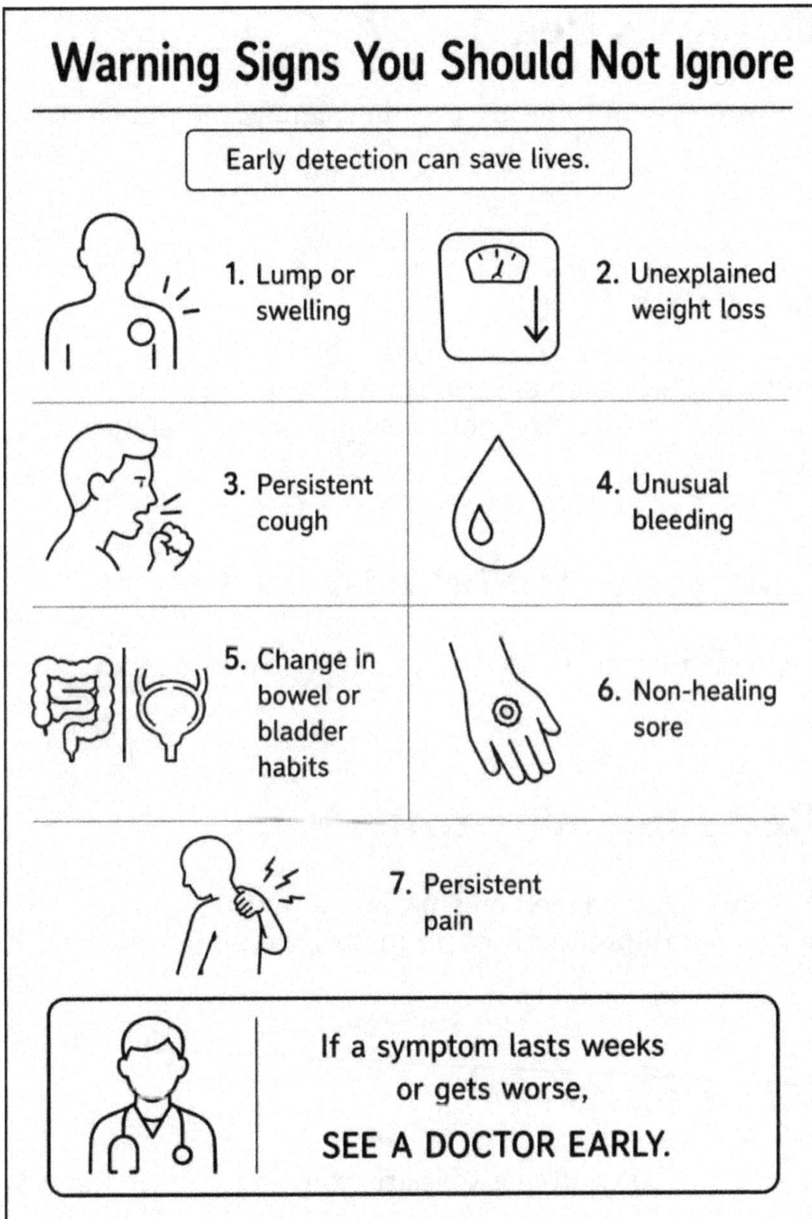
Warning Signs You Should Not Ignore
Early detection can save lives.
1. Lump or swelling
2. Unexplained weight loss
3. Persistent cough
4. Unusual bleeding
5. Change in bowel or bladder habits
6. Non-healing sore
7. Persistent pain
If a symptom lasts weeks or gets worse,
SEE A DOCTOR EARLY.

Doctor’s Pearl

Persistent symptoms are warning signals. Do not ignore them.

Myth vs Fact

Myth: If there is no pain, it cannot be serious.
Fact: Many cancers do not cause pain in early stages.

Common Mistake to Avoid

Delaying medical consultation due to fear or denial.

Red Flag Warning

Any unexplained bleeding, persistent lump, or long-lasting symptom requires prompt evaluation.

Key Points

- The body often gives early warning signs

- Persistence of symptoms is important
- Not all symptoms mean cancer, but they should not be ignored
- Some cancers are silent
- Early evaluation improves outcomes

Chapter Summary

Cancer may present with early warning signs, but these are often subtle and easily ignored. Symptoms such as unexplained weight loss, fatigue, lumps, bleeding, and changes in body habits should be taken seriously when they persist.

Early recognition and timely action can significantly improve outcomes.

Action Plan

- Pay attention to new or unusual symptoms
- Do not ignore persistent changes
- Seek medical advice when symptoms do not resolve
- Do not delay consultation due to fear
- Follow recommended screening guidelines

Bridge to Next Chapter

Recognizing symptoms is important, but many cancers can be detected even before symptoms appear.

In the next chapter, we will discuss screening and early detection, and how these tools can identify cancer at its earliest and most treatable stage.

CHAPTER 7: Screening and Early Detection: Finding Cancer Before It Causes Harm

Why Early Detection Changes Everything

If there is one concept in cancer care that truly saves lives, it is this.

Finding cancer early makes a major difference.

When cancer is detected early:

- It is usually smaller
- It has not spread
- Treatment is simpler
- The chances of success are much higher

When detected late, treatment becomes more complex and outcomes may not be as favorable.

Many cancers grow silently. You may feel completely well while changes are taking place inside the body.

Screening helps detect these changes before symptoms appear.

What Is Screening?

Screening means testing for cancer in people who do not have symptoms.

This is an important point.

Screening is not done because you feel unwell. It is done because you feel well, but we want to ensure that everything truly is normal.

Screening can:

- Detect cancer at an early stage
- Detect precancerous changes
- Prevent cancer in some cases

How Screening Helps Prevent Cancer

In some cancers, screening does more than detect disease. It can actually prevent it.

For example:

During a colonoscopy, small growths called polyps can be found and removed before they turn into cancer.

This is prevention in action.

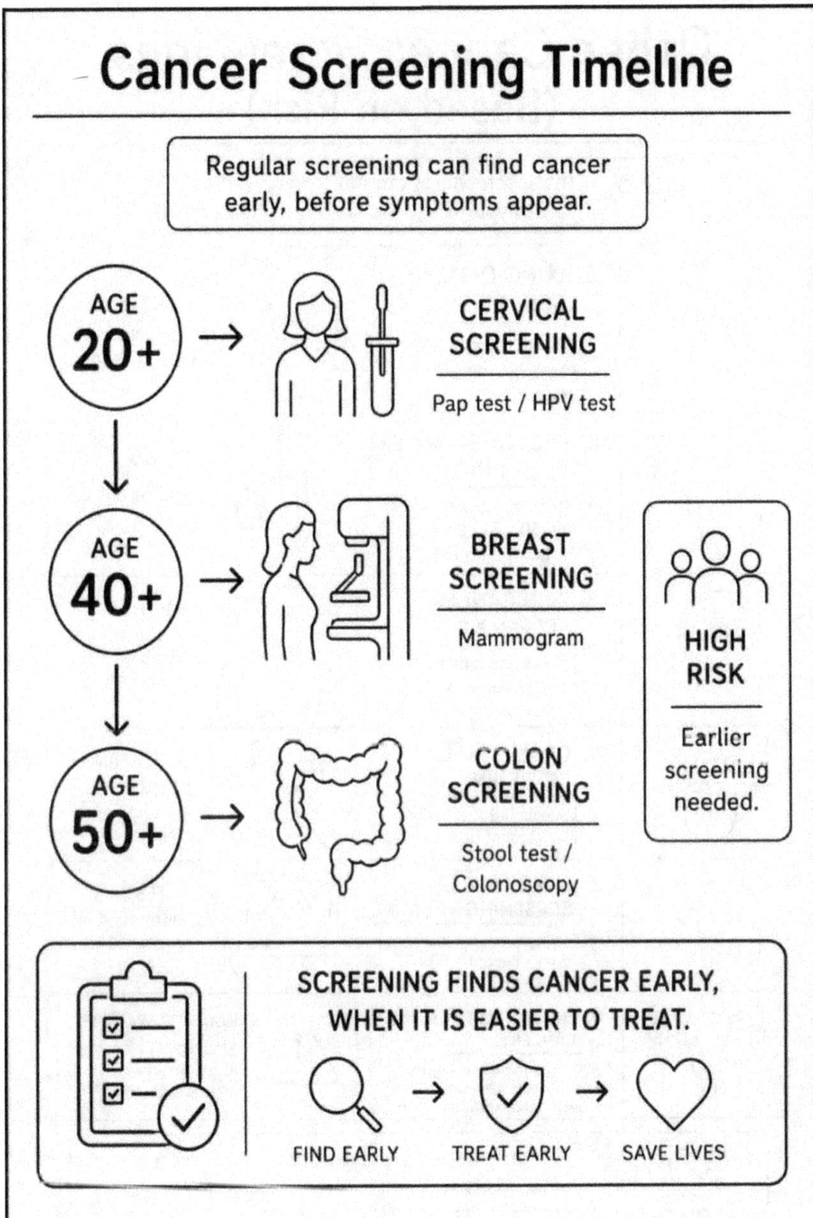
Cancer Screening Timeline
Regular screening can find cancer early, before symptoms appear.
AGE 20+
CERVICAL SCREENING
Pap test / HPV test
AGE 40+
BREAST SCREENING
Mammogram
AGE 50+
COLON SCREENING
Stool test / Colonoscopy
HIGH RISK
Earlier screening needed.
SCREENING FINDS CANCER EARLY, WHEN IT IS EASIER TO TREAT.
FIND EARLY
TREAT EARLY
SAVE LIVES

Other Cancer Screenings
(Based on Risk)

These screenings are not for everyone.
Talk to your doctor to see if you need them.

1. LUNG CANCER SCREENING

- For high-risk people, especially long-term smokers.

TEST: Low-dose CT scan

2. PROSTATE CANCER SCREENING

- For men, usually age 50 and above. Earlier if high risk.

TEST: PSA blood test

3. SKIN CANCER SCREENING

- No routine lab test.
- Check your skin regularly.

METHOD: Self-exam and doctor skin exam

4. ORAL CANCER SCREENING

- Especially for tobacco and alcohol users.

DONE DURING: Dental visits or routine examinations

5. LIVER CANCER SCREENING

- For high-risk people: chronic hepatitis B or C, or cirrhosis.

TEST: Ultrasound +/- blood test (AFP)

6. ENDOMETRIAL (UTERINE) CANCER

- No routine screening test.
- Important symptom: postmenopausal bleeding.

WHAT TO WATCH: Any vaginal bleeding after menopause — see a doctor.

Early detection saves lives.
Know your risk. Get the right screening.

Common Screening Tests You Should Know

Breast Cancer Screening

Mammography can detect breast cancer before it becomes a noticeable lump.

Regular screening improves early detection and outcomes.

Colon Cancer Screening

Options include:

- Colonoscopy
- Stool-based tests

Colonoscopy is particularly valuable because it can both detect and prevent cancer.

Cervical Cancer Screening

Pap test and HPV testing can detect early changes before cancer develops.

This is one of the most successful examples of cancer prevention.

Lung Cancer Screening

Low-dose CT scans are recommended for certain high-risk individuals, especially long-term smokers.

This can detect lung cancer at an earlier stage.

Prostate Cancer Screening

The PSA blood test may help detect prostate cancer.

However, screening decisions should be individualized after discussion with a doctor.

Who Should Get Screened?

Screening is not the same for everyone.

It depends on:

- Age
- Gender
- Family history
- Personal risk factors

For example:

- Individuals with a strong family history may need earlier screening
- Others may follow standard age-based recommendations

Your doctor can help decide what is appropriate for you.

Benefits of Screening

Screening offers several important benefits:

- Detects cancer early
- Improves chances of successful treatment
- May prevent cancer in certain cases
- Reduces the risk of advanced disease

These benefits are supported by strong medical evidence.

Limitations of Screening

It is important to understand that screening is not perfect.

Possible limitations include:

- False positives, where a test suggests cancer when it is not present
- False negatives, where cancer is missed
- Detection of slow-growing cancers that may not cause harm

These limitations do not reduce the value of screening, but they highlight the need for proper use and interpretation.

Why People Avoid Screening

Many people delay or avoid screening for simple reasons:

- They feel healthy
- They are afraid of the result
- They find it inconvenient

These concerns are understandable.

But avoiding screening may lead to missed opportunities for early detection.

A Practical Example

Consider two individuals.

One follows recommended screening and has a small cancer detected early, leading to effective treatment.

Another avoids screening and develops symptoms later, when the disease is more advanced.

The difference is timing.

Doctor's Pearl

Screening detects cancer early, when it is most treatable and sometimes preventable.

Myth vs Fact

Myth: If I feel fine, I do not need screening.
Fact: Many cancers do not cause symptoms in early stages.

Common Mistake to Avoid

Skipping recommended screening because you feel healthy.

Red Flag Warning

If you are eligible for screening and have not been tested, you are missing an important opportunity for early detection.

Key Points

- Screening detects cancer before symptoms appear
- Early detection improves outcomes
- Some screening tests can prevent cancer

- Screening recommendations vary by individual
- Screening has limitations but remains highly valuable

Chapter Summary

Screening and early detection are among the most effective tools in cancer care. By identifying disease at an early stage, screening allows for simpler and more effective treatment.

Regular screening, based on individual risk, is essential for long-term health.

Action Plan

- Know which screening tests apply to you
- Follow age-appropriate recommendations
- Discuss your personal risk with your doctor
- Do not delay screening because you feel well
- Stay consistent with follow-up

Bridge to Next Chapter

Now that you understand how cancer can be detected early, it is helpful to become familiar with the most common cancers.

In the next chapter, we will discuss common cancers that affect adults and what you should know about them in a practical way.

CHAPTER 8: Common Cancers Every Adult Should Understand

Why You Do Not Need to Know Everything, But You Should Know What Matters

Cancer is not a single disease. It includes many different types.

If you try to learn about every cancer, it can quickly become overwhelming.

But you do not need to know everything.

What you do need is a clear understanding of the cancers that are most common and most relevant in everyday life.

This chapter will focus on those.

The goal is simple.

To help you stay aware without becoming anxious.

Breast Cancer: Early Detection Makes a Big Difference

Breast cancer is one of the most common cancers in women.

What You Should Watch For

- A new lump in the breast
- Change in size or shape
- Skin dimpling or thickening
- Nipple discharge

What Helps

- Awareness of your own body
- Regular screening with mammography
- Early medical evaluation of any change

Breast cancer detected early is often highly treatable.

Prostate Cancer: Common and Often Silent

Prostate cancer is very common in men, especially with increasing age.

What You Should Watch For

- Difficulty passing urine
- Weak urine stream
- Frequent urination, especially at night

However, many men have no symptoms in early stages.

What Helps

- Discussion with your doctor about PSA testing

- Awareness of age-related risk

Some prostate cancers grow slowly, while others are more aggressive.

Lung Cancer: Strongly Linked to Smoking

Lung cancer remains one of the leading causes of cancer-related deaths.

Major Risk Factor

- Tobacco use

What You Should Watch For

- Persistent cough
- Blood in sputum
- Shortness of breath
- Chest pain

What Helps

- Avoiding tobacco
- Screening for high-risk individuals

Early detection can improve outcomes.

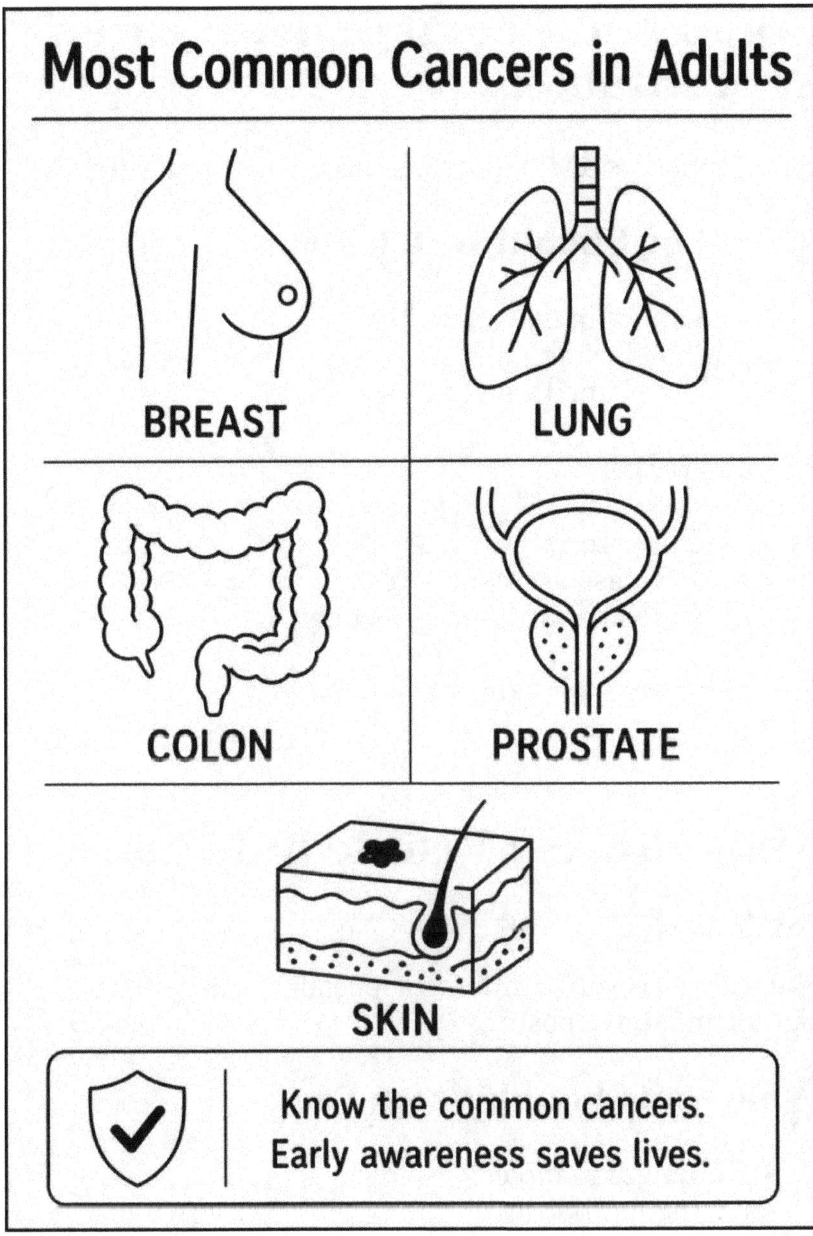
Most Common Cancers in Adults
BREAST
LUNG
COLON
PROSTATE
SKIN
Know the common cancers.
Early awareness saves lives.

Colon and Rectal Cancer: Often Preventable

Colon cancer is one of the most preventable cancers.

What You Should Watch For

- Changes in bowel habits
- Blood in stool
- Unexplained weight loss

What Helps

- Colonoscopy
- Stool-based screening tests
- Removal of precancerous polyps

Screening plays a major role in prevention.

Skin Cancer: Visible but Often Ignored

Skin cancer is very common, especially in people with significant sun exposure.

What You Should Watch For

- Changes in moles
- Irregular borders
- Variation in color
- Non-healing sores

What Helps

- Sun protection
- Regular skin checks

Early detection is usually straightforward.

Blood Cancers: A Different Pattern

Leukemia and lymphoma affect the blood and immune system.

What You Should Watch For

- Persistent fatigue
- Frequent infections
- Swollen lymph nodes
- Fever or night sweats

These cancers do not form solid lumps in the same way as other cancers.

Cancers Specific to Men and Women

Common in Women

- Cervical cancer

- Ovarian cancer
- Uterine cancer

Common in Men

- Testicular cancer

Each of these has specific symptoms and risk factors.

Awareness helps in early detection.

A Simple Pattern to Remember

Although cancers differ, some patterns are common:

- Risk increases with age
- Early stages often have no symptoms
- Screening improves detection
- Lifestyle influences risk

Keeping these patterns in mind simplifies a complex subject.

A Practical Example

Two individuals have similar risk factors.

One is aware of common cancers and follows screening.

The other ignores screening and symptoms.

Even if both develop cancer, the first individual is more likely to be diagnosed early and treated effectively.

Doctor's Pearl

Awareness of common cancers helps you act early and wisely.

Myth vs Fact

Myth: Cancer always shows clear symptoms early.
Fact: Many cancers develop silently and are detected through screening.

Common Mistake to Avoid

Ignoring routine screening because you feel well.

Red Flag Warning

Any persistent symptom related to a specific organ should be evaluated.

Key Points

- Cancer includes many different diseases
- Some cancers are more common than others
- Early stages often have no symptoms
- Screening is essential
- Awareness improves outcomes

Chapter Summary

Understanding common cancers allows you to focus on what truly matters. Each type has its own warning signs, but many share common patterns.

Awareness, screening, and timely action can significantly improve outcomes.

Action Plan

- Be aware of common cancers for your age and gender
- Follow recommended screening
- Pay attention to symptoms
- Seek medical advice for persistent changes
- Maintain a proactive approach to health

Bridge to Next Chapter

Now that you understand the common cancers, the next step is to understand how doctors confirm a diagnosis.

In the next chapter, we will walk through the process of cancer diagnosis in a clear and simple way.

CHAPTER 9: How Cancer Is Diagnosed: From Suspicion to Certainty

It Begins with a Concern, Not a Conclusion

In real life, cancer diagnosis does not usually begin with certainty.

It begins with a concern.

A symptom that does not go away.
An abnormal finding on a routine test.
A screening result that needs further evaluation.

At this stage, nothing is confirmed.

This is important to understand.

A concern is not a diagnosis.

Many findings that raise suspicion turn out to be non-cancerous. The purpose of evaluation is to move step by step toward clarity.

The First Step: Careful Listening and Examination

When you see a doctor, the process begins with understanding your story.

Your doctor will ask:

- What symptoms you have noticed
- When they started
- Whether they are changing
- Your medical history
- Your family history

This is followed by a physical examination.

This step may seem simple, but it provides valuable information.

Blood Tests: Helpful but Not Final

Blood tests are often part of the initial evaluation.

They may:

- Assess overall health
- Check organ function
- Detect certain markers

Some cancers produce substances called tumor markers.

However, it is important to remember:

- Tumor markers are not specific

- They can be elevated in non-cancer conditions
- They may be normal even if cancer is present

Blood tests alone cannot confirm cancer.

Imaging Tests: Looking Inside the Body

Imaging allows doctors to see what is happening inside the body.

Common tests include:

- X-ray
- Ultrasound
- CT scan
- MRI
- PET scan

Each test has a specific purpose.

Imaging can identify abnormalities, but it usually cannot confirm whether a growth is cancer.

Biopsy: The Most Important Step

A biopsy is the key step in diagnosing cancer.

It involves taking a small sample of tissue from the suspicious area and examining it under a microscope.

This is the only way to confirm cancer.

Types of biopsy include:

- Needle biopsy
- Surgical biopsy
- Endoscopic biopsy

The method depends on the location of the abnormality.

Biopsy is a safe and essential procedure.

The Pathology Report: Understanding the Details

After a biopsy, the tissue is examined by a pathologist.

The pathology report provides important information:

- Whether cancer is present
- The type of cancer
- Characteristics of the cancer cells

This report guides further evaluation and treatment.

Your doctor will help explain these details in simple terms.

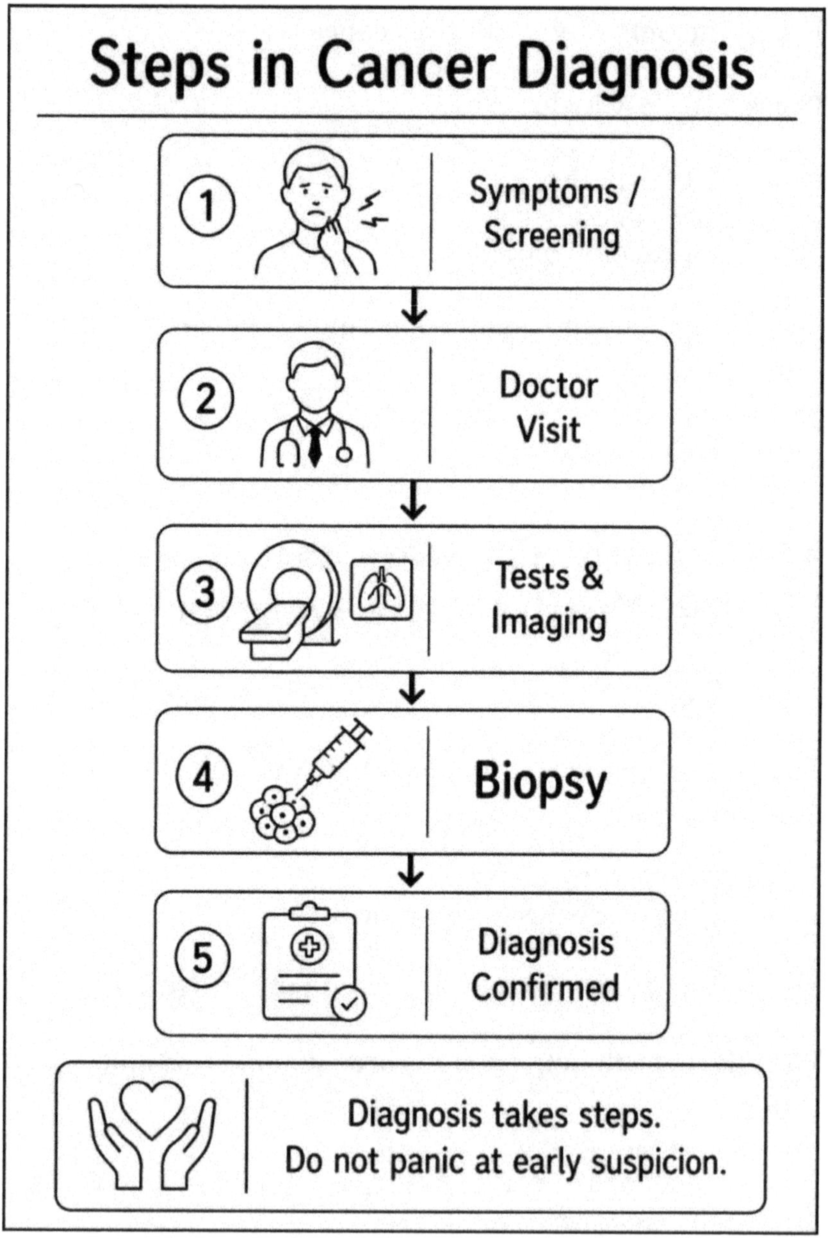
Steps in Cancer Diagnosis
1
Symptoms / Screening
2
Doctor Visit
3
Tests & Imaging
4
Biopsy
5
Diagnosis Confirmed
Diagnosis takes steps.
Do not panic at early suspicion.

Putting the Information Together

A diagnosis is not based on one test.

It is based on a combination of:

- Symptoms
- Physical examination
- Blood tests
- Imaging
- Biopsy results

Each step adds clarity.

Only after all these steps are complete can a diagnosis be confirmed.

Why the Process Takes Time

Waiting for results can be stressful.

Patients often want immediate answers.

But careful evaluation takes time.

Rushing the process can lead to errors.

A step-by-step approach ensures accuracy.

A Practical Example

A person develops a persistent cough.

An X-ray shows an abnormal area. A CT scan provides more detail. A biopsy confirms the diagnosis.

Each step is necessary.

Doctor's Pearl

A biopsy confirms cancer. Until then, it remains a possibility, not a certainty.

Myth vs Fact

Myth: A biopsy causes cancer to spread.
Fact: Biopsy is safe and does not cause cancer spread in routine practice.

Common Mistake to Avoid

Assuming a diagnosis without proper confirmation.

Red Flag Warning

Do not delay recommended tests or biopsy once advised.

Key Points

- Diagnosis begins with suspicion
- Blood tests and imaging provide clues
- Biopsy confirms cancer
- Multiple steps are required
- A careful approach is essential

Chapter Summary

Cancer diagnosis is a structured process that moves from suspicion to confirmation. It involves clinical evaluation, imaging, laboratory tests, and biopsy.

Each step plays an important role in ensuring an accurate diagnosis and guiding treatment decisions.

Action Plan

- Seek medical advice for concerning symptoms
- Follow recommended tests
- Do not panic if cancer is suspected
- Understand the importance of biopsy
- Ask questions and seek clarity

Bridge to Next Chapter

Once cancer is diagnosed, the next important question is:

How serious is it?

In the next chapter, we will explain stage, grade, and prognosis in a simple and practical way.

CHAPTER 10: Understanding Stage, Grade, and Prognosis: What It Really Means for You

After Diagnosis: The Questions That Naturally Follow

Once cancer is confirmed, the focus quickly shifts.

Patients begin to ask:

- How serious is it?
- Has it spread?
- What does this mean for my future?

These are important and reasonable questions.

The answers come from understanding three key concepts:

Stage, grade, and prognosis.

These may sound technical at first, but they can be understood clearly when explained step by step.

Stage: How Far Has the Cancer Spread?

Stage describes the extent of cancer in the body.

It tells us:

- The size of the tumor
- Whether it has spread to nearby tissues
- Whether it has reached distant organs

In simple terms:

- **Stage 1**: Cancer is small and confined
- **Stage 2**: Cancer is larger or beginning to spread locally
- **Stage 3**: Cancer has spread to nearby lymph nodes or tissues
- **Stage 4**: Cancer has spread to distant parts of the body

The earlier the stage, the better the chances for successful treatment.

Another Way to Understand Stage

Doctors may also use broader terms:

- **Localized**: Limited to the original site
- **Regional**: Spread to nearby areas
- **Metastatic**: Spread to distant organs

These terms help simplify the concept.

Understanding Cancer Stages

STAGE 1

Small, Local

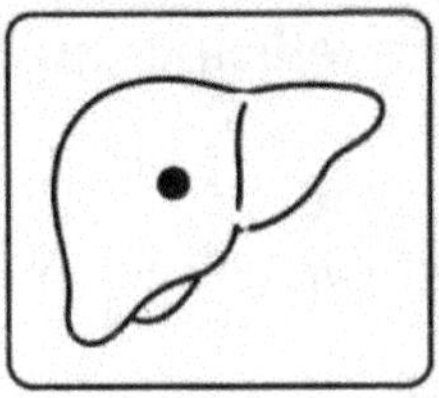

→ Cancer is small and confined to the original organ.

STAGE 2

Larger, Still Local

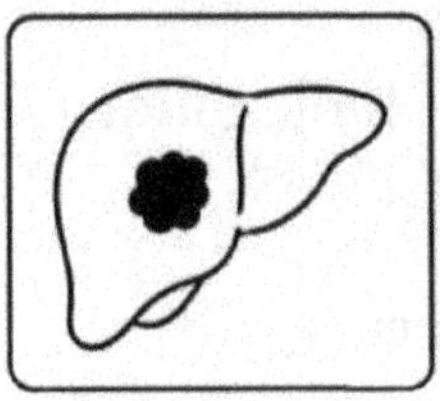

→ Cancer is larger but still in the original organ.

STAGE 3

Nearby Spread

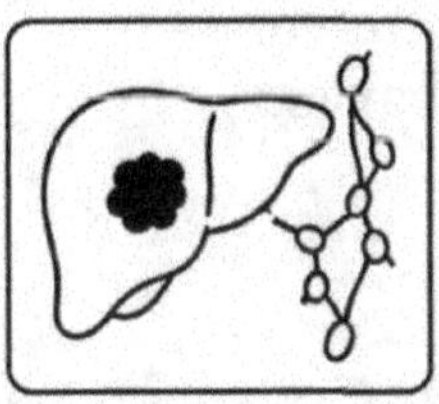

→ Cancer has spread to nearby lymph nodes or tissues.

STAGE 4

Distant Spread

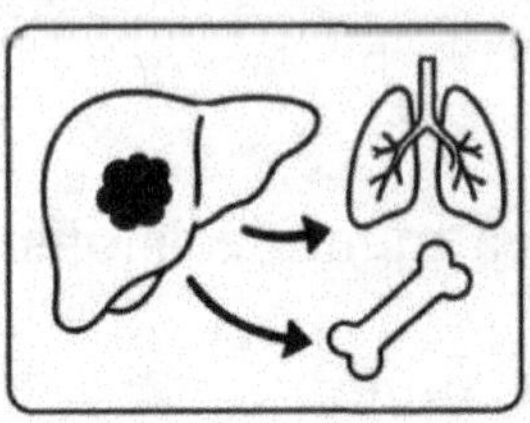

→ Cancer has spread to distant organs such as lungs, liver, bones, or others.

Earlier stage means easier treatment and better outcomes.

Grade: How Aggressive Is the Cancer?

Grade refers to how cancer cells look under the microscope.

It gives an idea of how fast the cancer may grow.

- **Low grade**: Cells look more like normal cells and usually grow slowly
- **High grade**: Cells look abnormal and tend to grow more quickly

A simple way to remember:

Stage tells you where the cancer is.
Grade tells you how it behaves.

Why Stage and Grade Are Important

These factors guide treatment decisions.

They help doctors determine:

- The type of treatment needed
- The intensity of treatment
- The likely course of the disease

For example:

- Early-stage, low-grade cancer may need less aggressive treatment
- Advanced or high-grade cancer may require more intensive therapy

---

Prognosis: What to Expect

Prognosis refers to the expected outcome of the disease.

It is based on several factors:

- Stage
- Grade
- Type of cancer
- Overall health
- Response to treatment

It is important to understand that prognosis is an estimate.

It is not a fixed prediction.

Understanding Survival Statistics

You may hear terms such as "5-year survival rate."

These are based on studies of large groups of patients.

It is important to interpret them carefully:

- They apply to groups, not individuals
- They may reflect older treatment data
- They cannot predict your personal outcome

Your situation is unique.

Why Outcomes Differ Between Individuals

Even with the same diagnosis, outcomes can vary.

This depends on:

- Individual biology
- General health
- Response to treatment
- Advances in medical care

Medicine is not only about numbers. It is about personalized care.

Questions You Should Ask Your Doctor

Clear communication helps reduce anxiety.

Consider asking:

- What stage is my cancer?
- What does the grade mean?
- Has the cancer spread?
- What are my treatment options?
- What is the goal of treatment?

Understanding your condition allows better decisions.

A Practical Example

Two patients are diagnosed with the same type of cancer.

One is diagnosed at an early stage and treated successfully.

Another is diagnosed at a later stage and requires more complex treatment.

The stage plays a major role in this difference.

Doctor's Pearl

Stage tells you how far cancer has spread. Grade tells you how aggressive it is.

Myth vs Fact

Myth: A higher stage means there is no hope.
Fact: Even advanced cancers can often be treated and controlled.

Common Mistake to Avoid

Focusing only on statistics instead of your individual situation.

Red Flag Warning

Do not make decisions based on incomplete information. Always discuss details with your doctor.

Key Points

- Stage describes spread
- Grade describes behavior
- Prognosis is an estimate
- Statistics apply to groups, not individuals
- Understanding helps guide treatment

Chapter Summary

Stage, grade, and prognosis are essential in understanding cancer. They provide information about how far the disease has progressed and how it may behave.

This understanding helps guide treatment decisions and reduces uncertainty.

Action Plan

- Ask your doctor to explain stage and grade clearly
- Do not rely only on statistics
- Focus on your individual condition
- Stay informed without unnecessary anxiety
- Maintain open communication with your care team

Bridge to Next Chapter

Now that you understand the seriousness of the diagnosis, the next step is to know what to do.

In the next chapter, we will discuss the practical steps to take after a cancer diagnosis in a clear and organized way.

CHAPTER 11: What To Do First After a Cancer Diagnosis: A Clear and Practical Path Forward

The First Moments: Pause Before You React

Hearing the word cancer can feel overwhelming.

The mind moves quickly. Thoughts race ahead.

"What will happen now?"
"Do I need treatment immediately?"
"Am I running out of time?"

In this moment, the most important advice I give my patients is simple.

Pause. Understand. Then act.

In most situations, you do not need to make decisions within hours. You usually have time to understand your condition and plan your next steps carefully.

A calm approach leads to better decisions.

Step One: Understand Your Diagnosis Clearly

Before anything else, you must understand what has been diagnosed.

Ask your doctor:

- What type of cancer is this?
- What stage is it?
- Has it spread?
- What is the goal of treatment?

If something is unclear, ask again.

Clear understanding is the foundation of good decision-making.

Step Two: Organize Your Medical Information

When everything feels uncertain, organization brings clarity.

Keep all your medical records in one place:

- Biopsy reports
- Imaging reports such as CT or MRI
- Blood test results
- Consultation notes

This helps when:

- You meet new specialists
- You seek a second opinion
- You review your treatment plan

It also gives you a sense of control.

Step Three: Build the Right Care Team

Cancer care is usually provided by a team.

This may include:

- A medical oncologist
- A surgeon
- A radiation specialist
- Your primary care doctor

Choosing the right team matters.

Look for:

- Experience with your condition
- Clear communication
- Willingness to answer questions

You should feel comfortable and confident with your care team.

Step Four: Consider a Second Opinion

A second opinion is often helpful.

It does not mean you doubt your doctor.

It means you want to confirm the diagnosis and treatment plan.

A second opinion can:

- Reinforce your confidence
- Offer additional options
- Provide reassurance

Most doctors support this step.

Step Five: Understand Your Treatment Plan

Before starting treatment, take time to understand it.

Ask:

- What treatment is recommended?
- Why is it recommended?
- What are the benefits and risks?
- What side effects may occur?

When you understand the plan, you feel more prepared and less anxious.

Step Six: Bring Support to Your Appointments

Medical discussions can involve a lot of information.

Having a trusted person with you can help.

They can:

- Listen carefully
- Help ask questions
- Remember important details

This support is both practical and emotional.

Step Seven: Plan Practical Matters Early

Cancer treatment can affect daily life.

It is helpful to plan ahead:

- Arrange time away from work if needed
- Plan transportation to appointments
- Organize help at home
- Review insurance and financial matters

Addressing these early reduces stress later.

Step Eight: Be Careful with Information Sources

Information is easily available, but not all of it is reliable.

Too much information can create confusion.

Focus on:

- Your doctor's advice
- Trusted medical sources

Avoid jumping between multiple opinions.

Step Nine: Focus on What You Can Control

There are many things you cannot control after a diagnosis.

But there are important things you can control:

- Your understanding
- Your decisions
- Your lifestyle
- Your attitude

Focusing on these areas gives you strength.

A Practical Example

One patient reacts with panic, searches multiple sources, and delays decisions.

Another takes a structured approach, understands the diagnosis, and begins treatment with clarity.

The difference is not the disease.

It is the approach.

Doctor's Pearl

A calm, organized approach after diagnosis leads to better decisions and better outcomes.

Myth vs Fact

Myth: Treatment decisions must be made immediately.
Fact: In most cases, there is time to understand and plan properly.

Common Mistake to Avoid

Making rushed decisions without full understanding.

Red Flag Warning

Do not delay necessary treatment for long periods while seeking multiple opinions.

Key Points

- Do not panic after diagnosis
- Understand your condition clearly
- Organize your medical information
- Choose the right care team
- Consider a second opinion
- Plan practical matters early

Chapter Summary

A cancer diagnosis is a major life event, but the steps that follow are equally important. Taking a calm and organized approach helps reduce anxiety and leads to better decisions.

Understanding your diagnosis, choosing the right care team, and planning ahead are essential parts of effective care.

Action Plan

- Take time to understand your diagnosis
- Ask clear questions
- Keep your medical records organized
- Consider a second opinion
- Bring support to appointments
- Plan practical needs early

Bridge to Next Chapter

Now that you know what to do after diagnosis, the next step is to understand treatment options.

In the next chapter, we will explain the main types of cancer treatment in a clear and practical way.

CHAPTER 12: Cancer Treatment: Understanding Your Options with Clarity and Confidence

Moving from Diagnosis to Treatment

Once the diagnosis is confirmed, attention naturally turns to treatment.

This is often the stage where anxiety increases again.

Patients commonly ask:

- What treatment will I need?
- Will it be painful?
- What are my chances?

These concerns are completely understandable.

In my experience, much of this fear comes from uncertainty. When patients clearly understand their treatment options, they feel more prepared and more in control.

Cancer treatment today is more advanced, more precise, and more personalized than ever before.

First, Understand the Goal of Treatment

Before discussing specific treatments, it is important to understand the goal.

Cancer treatment is not the same for every patient.

The goal may be:

- **Cure**: To completely eliminate the cancer
- **Control**: To slow or reduce the growth of cancer
- **Relief**: To reduce symptoms and improve comfort

Knowing the goal helps you understand why a particular treatment is recommended.

Surgery: Removing the Cancer

Surgery is one of the most effective treatments, especially when cancer is localized.

When It Is Used

- When the tumor can be removed completely
- When cancer is confined to one area

What It Involves

The surgeon removes the tumor along with a small margin of surrounding tissue.

Important Points

- It may require a hospital stay
- Recovery time varies
- Additional treatment may be needed

In many early cancers, surgery can be curative.

Radiation Therapy: Targeted Treatment

Radiation therapy uses high-energy rays to destroy cancer cells.

How It Works

It damages the DNA of cancer cells, preventing them from growing.

When It Is Used

- Before surgery to shrink a tumor
- After surgery to destroy remaining cells
- As a main treatment in certain cases

What to Expect

- Usually given over several sessions
- The procedure itself is painless
- Side effects depend on the area treated

Radiation therapy is precise and carefully planned.

CANCER TREATMENT OPTIONS

Treatment is planned based on the type, stage, and your health.

1 SURGERY

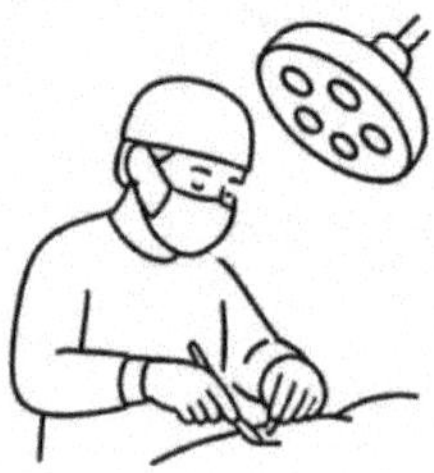

Remove cancer from the body.

2 CHEMOTHERAPY

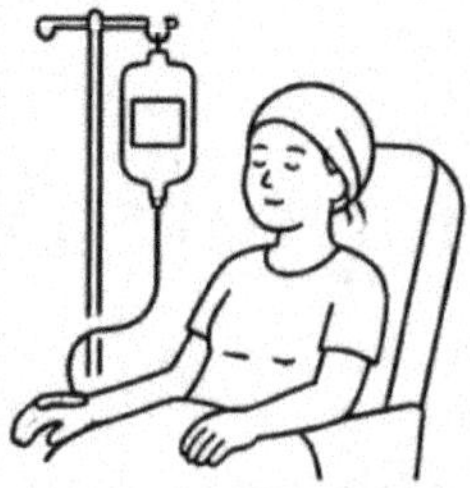

Use medicine to kill cancer cells.

3 RADIATION THERAPY

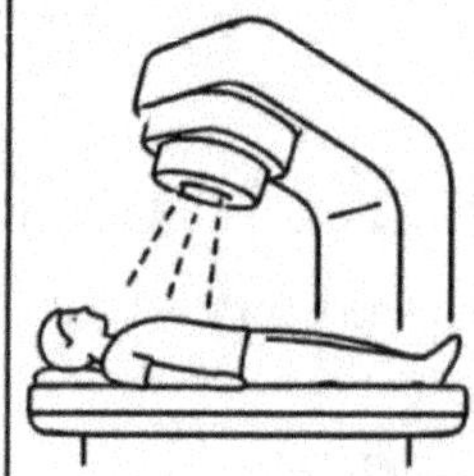

Use high-energy rays to kill cancer cells.

4 IMMUNOTHERAPY

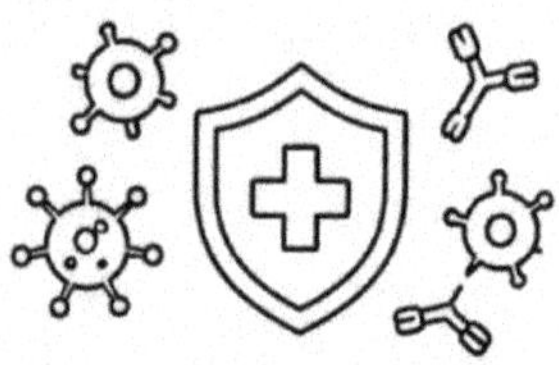

Help your immune system fight cancer.

5 TARGETED THERAPY

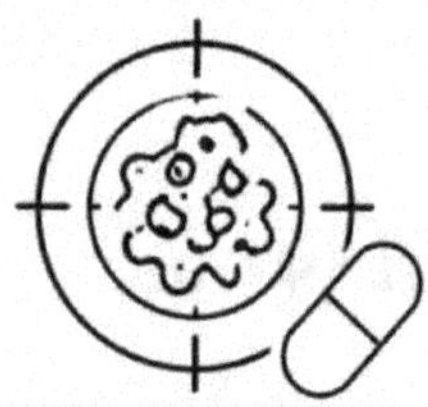

Use drugs that target specific changes in cancer cells.

Often, a combination of treatments works best.

Your treatment is personal.
Your care team is with you every step.

Chemotherapy: Treating the Whole Body

Chemotherapy uses drugs that travel through the bloodstream to destroy cancer cells.

When It Is Used

- When cancer has spread
- When there is a risk of spread
- Along with other treatments

What to Expect

- Given in cycles
- May cause side effects such as fatigue, nausea, or hair loss
- Side effects are often manageable

Chemotherapy remains a powerful treatment option.

Immunotherapy: Helping the Body Fight Cancer

Immunotherapy is one of the most important recent advances.

How It Works

It strengthens the immune system so it can recognize and attack cancer cells.

When It Is Used

- In certain cancers
- Often when other treatments are less effective

What to Expect

- Given as injections or infusions
- Side effects are different from chemotherapy
- Can be highly effective in selected patients

Targeted Therapy: Precision Medicine

Targeted therapy focuses on specific changes in cancer cells.

How It Works

It blocks signals that cancer cells need to grow.

Advantages

- More precise action
- Often fewer side effects

Limitations

- Works only for certain cancers

This is part of personalized cancer treatment.

Hormone Therapy

Some cancers depend on hormones to grow.

Examples

- Breast cancer
- Prostate cancer

How It Works

Hormone therapy blocks or reduces the effect of these hormones.

Combination Treatment: A Coordinated Plan

Many patients receive more than one type of treatment.

Examples include:

- Surgery followed by chemotherapy
- Radiation combined with chemotherapy

This approach improves effectiveness.

Treatment is carefully planned based on individual needs.

Understanding Side Effects

All treatments may cause side effects, but not everyone experiences them in the same way.

Common side effects include:

- Fatigue
- Nausea
- Hair loss
- Skin changes

Important points:

- Side effects vary from person to person
- Many can be managed effectively
- Treatment can be adjusted if needed

Fear of side effects should not prevent appropriate treatment.

A Practical Example

One patient starts treatment early and follows a well-planned approach.

Another delays treatment due to fear.

The first patient often has better outcomes.

The difference is timely action and understanding.

Doctor's Pearl

Cancer treatment is individualized. The same disease may be treated differently in different patients.

Myth vs Fact

Myth: Cancer treatment is always unbearable.
Fact: Many treatments are well tolerated, and side effects can be managed.

Common Mistake to Avoid

Delaying treatment because of fear without understanding the benefits.

Red Flag Warning

Avoid relying on unproven alternative therapies instead of medical treatment.

Key Points

- Treatment goals may be cure, control, or relief
- Surgery, radiation, and chemotherapy are main treatments
- Newer treatments include immunotherapy and targeted therapy
- Combination therapy is common
- Side effects are often manageable

Chapter Summary

Cancer treatment involves multiple approaches, each chosen based on the type and stage of cancer. Modern treatment is more personalized and more effective than in the past.

Understanding these options helps reduce fear and supports better decision-making.

Action Plan

- Understand the goal of your treatment
- Ask about all available options
- Learn about possible side effects
- Follow your treatment plan carefully
- Avoid unproven alternatives

Bridge to Next Chapter

Now that you understand the main treatment options, let us take a closer look at one of the most common approaches.

In the next chapter, we will discuss surgery for cancer and what you can expect before, during, and after the procedure.

CHAPTER 13: Surgery for Cancer: What It Means and What to Expect

Understanding Surgery Without Fear

When patients hear that surgery is needed, the reaction is often immediate.

"Is it serious?"
"Will I recover?"
"What will happen to me?"

These concerns are completely natural.

In my experience, fear of surgery usually comes from not knowing what to expect. When patients understand the purpose and process, their confidence improves.

Surgery is not something to fear blindly.

It is often the most direct and effective way to remove cancer.

Why Surgery Is Recommended

Surgery is most useful when cancer is localized.

This means:

- The tumor is confined to one area
- It can be removed completely

In such cases, surgery may offer the best chance for cure.

Surgery may also be used to:

- Reduce tumor size
- Relieve symptoms such as pain or blockage
- Improve the effectiveness of other treatments

The role of surgery depends on each individual case.

Types of Cancer Surgery

Not all surgeries have the same purpose.

Curative Surgery

The goal is to remove all cancer. This is often possible in early stages.

Debulking Surgery

Removes as much tumor as possible when complete removal is not feasible.

Palliative Surgery

Focuses on relieving symptoms and improving comfort.

Understanding the purpose of your surgery helps set expectations.

Modern Surgical Techniques

Surgery has advanced significantly.

Open Surgery

Traditional method with a larger incision.

Minimally Invasive Surgery

Includes laparoscopic and robotic techniques using small incisions.

Benefits of Minimally Invasive Surgery

- Less pain
- Shorter hospital stay
- Faster recovery

Not all patients are suitable for these methods, but when possible, they offer clear advantages.

Preparing for Surgery

Preparation plays an important role in recovery.

Before surgery:

- Follow your doctor's instructions carefully
- Inform your doctor about all medications
- Stop smoking if applicable
- Maintain good nutrition
- Arrange support at home

Good preparation helps improve outcomes.

What Happens During Surgery

During the operation:

- You will be given anesthesia
- The surgeon will remove the tumor
- A margin of surrounding tissue is often removed
- Nearby lymph nodes may also be examined

You will not feel pain during the procedure.

The surgical team monitors your condition continuously.

Recovery After Surgery

Recovery depends on the type of surgery.

You may experience:

- Pain or discomfort
- Fatigue
- Temporary limitations in activity

Your doctor will guide you on:

- Wound care
- Activity level
- Follow-up visits

Recovery is gradual, and most patients return to their normal routine over time.

Risks and Complications

All surgeries carry some risk.

Possible risks include:

- Infection
- Bleeding
- Reaction to anesthesia

Serious complications are less common, especially with experienced surgical teams.

Understanding risks helps you prepare, but should not create unnecessary fear.

When Surgery May Not Be Suitable

In some cases, surgery may not be the best option.

This may happen when:

- Cancer has spread widely
- The tumor is in a difficult location
- Overall health makes surgery risky

In such situations, other treatments may be more appropriate.

A Practical Example

One patient has early-stage cancer and undergoes surgery that removes the tumor completely.

Another has advanced cancer where surgery is used to relieve symptoms.

In both cases, surgery plays an important role, but the goal is different.

Doctor's Pearl

When cancer is localized, surgery often offers the best chance for cure.

Myth vs Fact

Myth: Surgery causes cancer to spread.
Fact: Surgery is carefully performed and does not cause cancer spread.

Common Mistake to Avoid

Delaying recommended surgery due to fear.

Red Flag Warning

Do not postpone necessary surgery without discussing risks with your doctor.

Key Points

- Surgery is a key treatment for many cancers
- It is most effective when cancer is localized
- Different types of surgery serve different purposes
- Modern techniques improve safety and recovery
- Preparation and follow-up are essential

Chapter Summary

Surgery remains one of the most important tools in cancer treatment. It is often the best option for removing localized cancer and can also help manage symptoms.

Advances in surgical techniques have made procedures safer and recovery easier.

Action Plan

- Understand why surgery is recommended
- Follow all preparation instructions
- Arrange support for recovery
- Discuss risks and expectations
- Attend follow-up appointments

Bridge to Next Chapter

Surgery is one part of treatment, but many patients also experience side effects from different therapies.

In the next chapter, we will discuss treatment side effects and how to manage them effectively.

CHAPTER 14: Side Effects of Cancer Treatment: What to Expect and How to Manage Them

Facing Side Effects with Understanding

When treatment begins, many patients worry about side effects.

This is understandable.

Stories from others, especially negative ones, often create fear. But what I have seen in practice is reassuring.

Most side effects today can be managed.

Not every patient experiences severe symptoms. Many go through treatment with mild or moderate effects that can be controlled with proper care.

The key is awareness and early action.

Why Side Effects Occur

Cancer treatments are designed to destroy cancer cells.

However, some normal cells in the body also divide quickly, such as:

- Cells in the hair
- Cells in the digestive system
- Cells in the bone marrow

Because of this, treatment may temporarily affect these normal cells.

The type and severity of side effects depend on:

- The type of treatment
- The dose and duration
- Your overall health

Fatigue: The Most Common Side Effect

Fatigue is very common.

This is not normal tiredness. It is a deeper sense of low energy that may not improve with rest.

What Helps

- Short periods of rest
- Light daily activity such as walking
- Regular sleep routine
- Balanced nutrition

Complete inactivity can make fatigue worse.

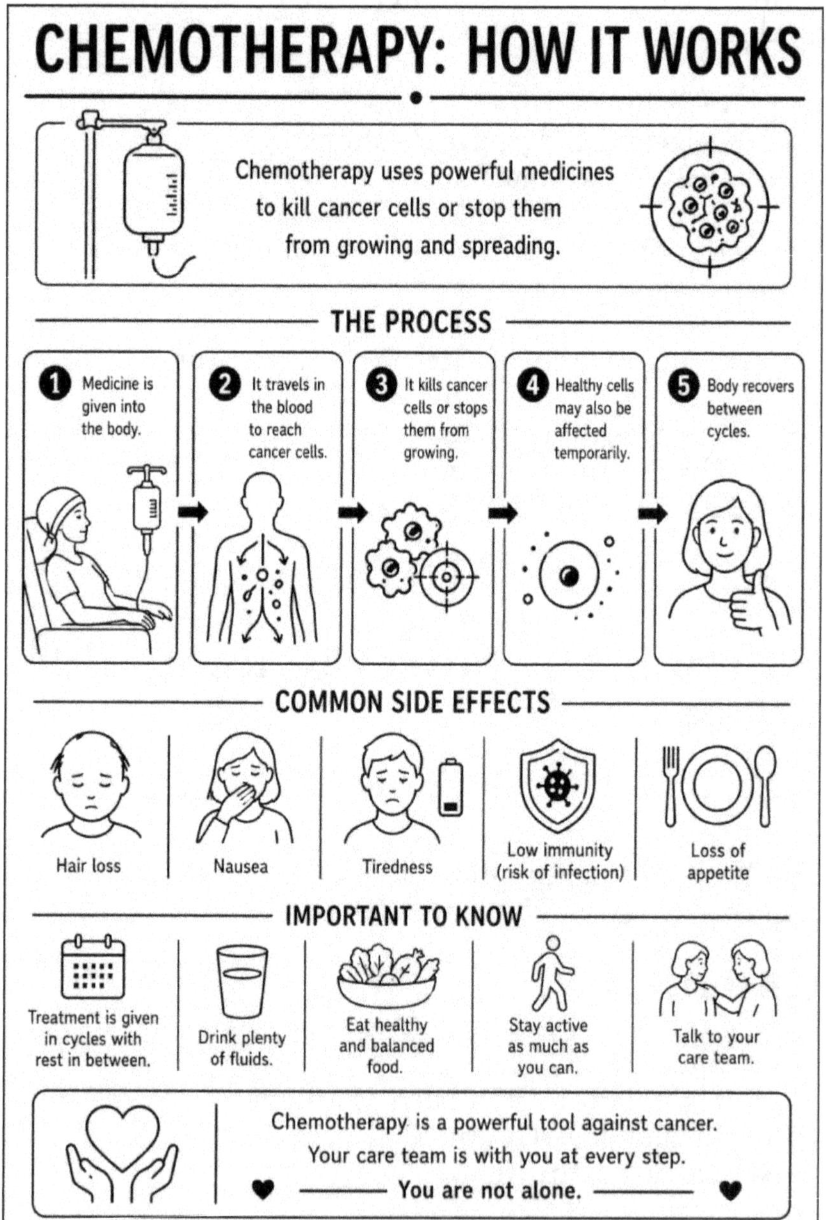
CHEMOTHERAPY: HOW IT WORKS
Chemotherapy uses powerful medicines to kill cancer cells or stop them from growing and spreading.
THE PROCESS
1 Medicine is given into the body.
2 It travels in the blood to reach cancer cells.
3 It kills cancer cells or stops them from growing.
4 Healthy cells may also be affected temporarily.
5 Body recovers between cycles.
COMMON SIDE EFFECTS
Hair loss
Nausea
Tiredness
Low immunity (risk of infection)
Loss of appetite
IMPORTANT TO KNOW
Treatment is given in cycles with rest in between.
Drink plenty of fluids.
Eat healthy and balanced food.
Stay active as much as you can.
Talk to your care team.
Chemotherapy is a powerful tool against cancer.
Your care team is with you at every step.
You are not alone.

Nausea and Digestive Changes

Some treatments affect the digestive system.

You may experience:

- Nausea
- Reduced appetite
- Changes in taste
- Constipation or diarrhea

Helpful Measures

- Eat small, frequent meals
- Stay well hydrated
- Use prescribed medications
- Choose simple, easy-to-digest foods

These symptoms are often manageable.

Hair Loss and Skin Changes

Certain treatments may cause hair loss.

This can be emotionally difficult, even though it is usually temporary.

Skin may also become:

- Dry
- Sensitive
- Irritated

Practical Care

- Use mild soaps
- Apply moisturizers
- Protect skin from sun exposure

Hair usually grows back after treatment ends.

Low Blood Counts and Infection Risk

Some treatments reduce white blood cells, increasing infection risk.

Warning Signs

- Fever
- Chills
- Persistent cough

Prevention Tips

- Maintain good hygiene
- Avoid contact with sick individuals
- Report symptoms early

Prompt attention is important.

Pain and Discomfort

Pain may occur due to:

- The cancer itself
- Treatment procedures

Pain can usually be controlled.

Management Options

- Medications
- Physical therapy
- Relaxation techniques

You should not feel that pain must be tolerated.

Emotional Side Effects

Treatment affects emotional well-being.

Patients may experience:

- Anxiety
- Sadness
- Irritability

These feelings are normal.

Ways to Cope

- Talk openly with family
- Maintain a routine
- Seek support if needed

Emotional care is as important as physical care.

Every Patient Is Different

Even with the same treatment:

- Some patients have minimal side effects
- Others may experience more symptoms

Do not compare your experience with others.

Your journey is unique.

When to Contact Your Doctor

Seek medical advice if you have:

- Fever
- Severe nausea or vomiting
- Uncontrolled pain
- Sudden worsening of symptoms

Early communication helps prevent complications.

A Practical Example

One patient reports side effects early and receives timely care.

Another ignores symptoms.

The first patient recovers more smoothly.

The difference is early action.

Doctor's Pearl

Most side effects can be controlled when addressed early.

Myth vs Fact

Myth: Cancer treatment always causes severe suffering.
Fact: Many side effects are manageable with modern care.

Common Mistake to Avoid

Ignoring symptoms or delaying communication with your doctor.

Red Flag Warning

Fever during treatment requires immediate medical attention.

Key Points

- Side effects occur because normal cells are affected
- Fatigue is the most common symptom
- Digestive issues, hair loss, and infection risk are common
- Emotional health is important
- Early reporting improves outcomes

Chapter Summary

Side effects are a common part of cancer treatment, but they are usually manageable. Understanding what to expect helps reduce fear and allows patients to take an active role in their care.

Modern cancer care focuses on both treating the disease and maintaining quality of life.

Action Plan

- Learn about possible side effects
- Report symptoms early
- Follow medical advice
- Maintain good nutrition and hydration
- Take care of emotional health
- Seek support when needed

Bridge to Next Chapter

Managing side effects is important, but daily living during treatment also plays a key role.

In the next chapter, we will discuss how to live well during and after treatment, focusing on practical steps for maintaining strength and well-being.

CHAPTER 15: Living Well During and After Treatment: Practical Steps for Strength and Recovery

Life Does Not Stop During Treatment

When treatment begins, many patients feel that life has come to a pause.

Everything seems to revolve around appointments, medications, and test results.

But I want you to understand something important.

Life does not stop during treatment.

It changes, yes. Your routine may slow down. Your energy may vary from day to day. But how you live each day still matters greatly.

In fact, your daily habits can support your treatment and improve your recovery.

Nutrition: Supporting Your Body from Within

During treatment, eating may become difficult.

You may notice:

- Reduced appetite
- Changes in taste
- Occasional nausea

Even then, nutrition remains essential.

Practical Approach

- Eat small, frequent meals
- Include protein in your diet
- Stay well hydrated
- Choose simple, freshly prepared foods

Avoid extreme diets. Focus on balance and consistency.

If eating becomes difficult, discuss it with your doctor. Support is available.

Physical Activity: Keep Moving, Gently

Many patients believe complete rest is best.

Rest is important, but too much inactivity can lead to:

- Weakness
- Loss of muscle strength
- Increased fatigue

Benefits of Light Activity

- Improves energy
- Maintains strength
- Supports emotional health

Simple Activities

- Short daily walks
- Gentle stretching
- Light household tasks

The goal is not intensity. It is regular movement.

Sleep and Rest: A Foundation for Healing

Good sleep supports recovery.

However, treatment and stress can disturb sleep patterns.

Helpful Habits

- Maintain a regular sleep schedule
- Keep your sleeping area calm and comfortable
- Avoid heavy meals before bedtime
- Limit screen time at night

Short rest periods during the day can help, but excessive daytime sleep may affect nighttime sleep.

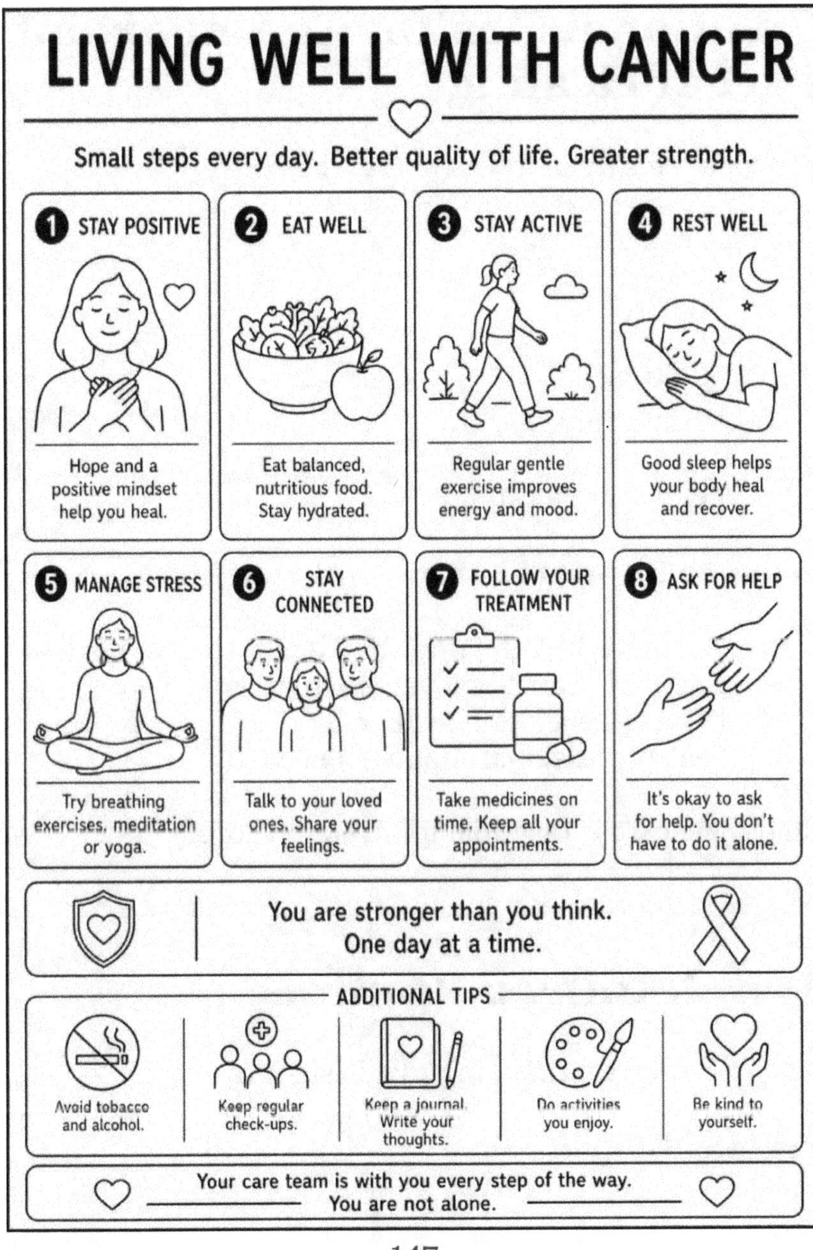
LIVING WELL WITH CANCER
Small steps every day. Better quality of life. Greater strength.
1 STAY POSITIVE
Hope and a positive mindset help you heal.
2 EAT WELL
Eat balanced, nutritious food. Stay hydrated.
3 STAY ACTIVE
Regular gentle exercise improves energy and mood.
4 REST WELL
Good sleep helps your body heal and recover.
5 MANAGE STRESS
Try breathing exercises, meditation or yoga.
6 STAY CONNECTED
Talk to your loved ones. Share your feelings.
7 FOLLOW YOUR TREATMENT
Take medicines on time. Keep all your appointments.
8 ASK FOR HELP
It's okay to ask for help. You don't have to do it alone.
You are stronger than you think.
One day at a time.
ADDITIONAL TIPS
Avoid tobacco and alcohol.
Keep regular check-ups.
Keep a journal. Write your thoughts.
Do activities you enjoy.
Be kind to yourself.
Your care team is with you every step of the way.
You are not alone.

Emotional Health: An Important Part of Healing

Cancer affects the mind as well as the body.

You may experience:

- Anxiety
- Sadness
- Irritability
- Uncertainty

These feelings are natural.

Ways to Support Emotional Health

- Talk openly with family or friends
- Engage in calm, enjoyable activities
- Practice relaxation techniques
- Seek professional support if needed

Emotional care is essential for overall recovery.

Maintaining a Routine

A simple daily routine can provide stability.

Practical Tips

- Continue normal activities when possible
- Adjust based on your energy level
- Avoid overexertion
- Accept help when needed

Routine brings a sense of normal life during treatment.

Support from Family and Caregivers

Cancer affects not only the patient but also the family.

Support from loved ones is valuable, but caregivers also need support.

Balanced Approach

- Communicate openly
- Share responsibilities
- Recognize the needs of caregivers

Care is most effective when it is shared.

Life After Treatment: A Gradual Return

After treatment ends, many expect to feel "back to normal" quickly.

In reality, recovery takes time.

You may notice:

- Gradual improvement in energy
- Emotional adjustment
- Continued medical follow-up

Recovery is a process.

Be patient with yourself.

Reducing the Risk of Recurrence

After treatment, focus shifts to long-term health.

Helpful steps include:

- Maintaining a healthy lifestyle
- Attending follow-up visits
- Reporting new symptoms early

These actions support long-term well-being.

A Practical Example

One patient maintains balanced nutrition, stays active, and remains emotionally connected.

Another becomes inactive and isolated.

The difference in recovery and quality of life can be significant.

Doctor's Pearl

Small, consistent daily habits play a major role in recovery and quality of life.

Myth vs Fact

Myth: Complete rest is best during treatment.
Fact: Gentle activity and balanced living improve recovery.

Common Mistake to Avoid

Neglecting nutrition, activity, or emotional well-being.

Red Flag Warning

Persistent weakness, inability to eat, or emotional distress should be discussed with your doctor.

Key Points

- Life continues during treatment
- Nutrition supports healing
- Gentle activity improves strength
- Sleep is essential
- Emotional health matters
- Recovery takes time

Chapter Summary

Living well during and after cancer treatment plays a major role in recovery. Nutrition, physical activity, sleep, and emotional health all contribute to better outcomes.

Treatment addresses the disease, while lifestyle supports the body and mind.

Action Plan

- Eat small, balanced meals
- Stay hydrated
- Engage in light activity
- Maintain a regular sleep routine
- Support your emotional health
- Stay connected with loved ones
- Attend follow-up appointments

Bridge to Next Chapter

While many patients recover well, some situations require a different approach.

In the next chapter, we will discuss advanced cancer and the role of supportive care, focusing on comfort and quality of life.

CHAPTER 16: When Cancer Is Advanced: Care, Comfort, and Dignity

Facing a Difficult Reality with Honesty and Compassion

There are times when cancer cannot be completely cured.

This is one of the hardest conversations in medicine.

I have sat with many patients and families during these moments. The room becomes quiet. Questions become fewer, but deeper.

"What does this mean for me?"
"What can be done now?"

Let me say this clearly.

When cure is not possible, care does not stop.

In many ways, care becomes even more focused on what truly matters.

What Is Advanced Cancer?

Advanced cancer usually means:

- The disease has spread to other parts of the body, or
- It cannot be completely removed or cured

This does not mean that nothing can be done.

In many cases, treatment can still:

- Slow the growth of cancer
- Reduce symptoms
- Improve comfort
- Extend meaningful life

Every situation is different. The plan is always individualized.

A Shift in Goals: From Cure to Control and Comfort

In earlier stages, treatment focuses on cure.

In advanced stages, the focus often changes to:

- Controlling the disease
- Relieving symptoms
- Maintaining quality of life

This is not giving up.

It is a thoughtful and appropriate change in approach.

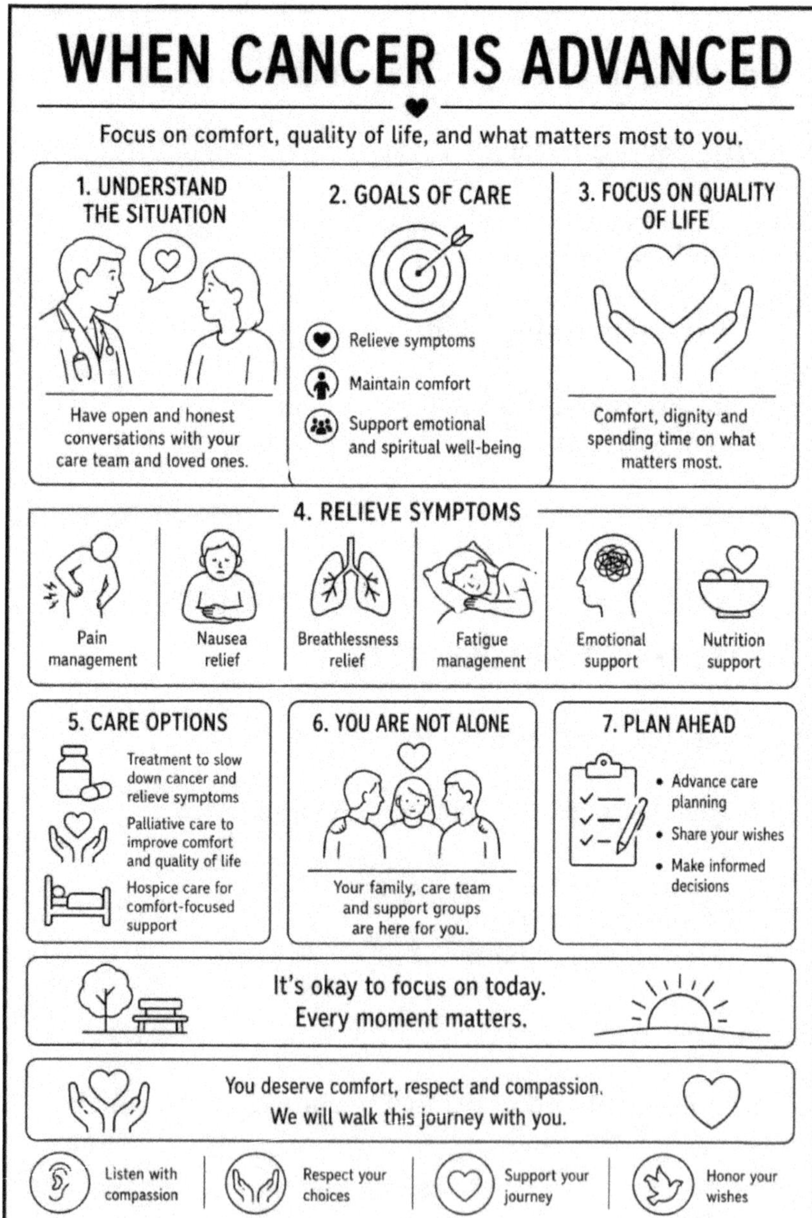
WHEN CANCER IS ADVANCED
Focus on comfort, quality of life, and what matters most to you.
1. UNDERSTAND THE SITUATION
Have open and honest conversations with your care team and loved ones.
2. GOALS OF CARE
Relieve symptoms
Maintain comfort
Support emotional and spiritual well-being
3. FOCUS ON QUALITY OF LIFE
Comfort, dignity and spending time on what matters most.
4. RELIEVE SYMPTOMS
Pain management
Nausea relief
Breathlessness relief
Fatigue management
Emotional support
Nutrition support
5. CARE OPTIONS
Treatment to slow down cancer and relieve symptoms
Palliative care to improve comfort and quality of life
Hospice care for comfort-focused support
6. YOU ARE NOT ALONE
Your family, care team and support groups are here for you.
7. PLAN AHEAD
• Advance care planning
• Share your wishes
• Make informed decisions
It's okay to focus on today. Every moment matters.
You deserve comfort, respect and compassion. We will walk this journey with you.
Listen with compassion
Respect your choices
Support your journey
Honor your wishes

Palliative Care: An Essential Part of Treatment

Palliative care is often misunderstood.

Many people think it is only for the final stage of life. That is not correct.

Palliative care is about improving quality of life at any stage of serious illness.

It includes:

- Pain control
- Symptom management
- Emotional support
- Assistance with daily challenges

Palliative care can be provided alongside active treatment.

Pain Management: Relief Is Possible

Pain is one of the greatest concerns for patients.

The important point is this.

In most cases, pain can be controlled.

Options include:

- Medications
- Targeted treatments such as radiation
- Specialized procedures

You should never feel that pain must be endured.

Open communication with your doctor is essential.

Managing Other Symptoms

Advanced cancer may cause:

- Shortness of breath
- Fatigue
- Loss of appetite
- Nausea

These symptoms can often be managed effectively.

The goal is always to improve comfort and maintain daily function.

Emotional Support: Caring for the Mind

Advanced illness affects emotional well-being.

Patients may experience:

- Fear
- Sadness
- Uncertainty
- Concern for family

These feelings are natural.

Support can come from:

- Family and friends
- Counseling
- Support groups

Emotional care is an essential part of overall care.

Supporting Family and Caregivers

Cancer affects the entire family.

Caregivers often carry a significant burden.

It is important to:

- Communicate openly
- Share responsibilities
- Recognize caregiver needs

Support should include both the patient and the family.

Hospice Care: Focus on Comfort

Hospice care is considered when the focus shifts fully to comfort rather than active treatment.

It provides:

- Pain and symptom control
- Emotional and spiritual support
- Assistance for family members

The goal is to maintain dignity and comfort.

Respecting Personal Wishes

Every patient has personal values and preferences.

It is important to discuss:

- Treatment choices
- Living arrangements
- End-of-life wishes

These conversations may be difficult, but they bring clarity and peace.

A Practical Example

One patient receives early palliative care, with good symptom control and strong support.

Another delays supportive care and experiences unnecessary discomfort.

The difference lies in planning and communication.

Doctor's Pearl

When cure is not possible, comfort, dignity, and quality of life become the most important goals.

Myth vs Fact

Myth: Palliative care means giving up.
Fact: Palliative care improves quality of life and can be started early.

Common Mistake to Avoid

Delaying supportive care due to misunderstanding.

Red Flag Warning

Uncontrolled pain or severe symptoms should be addressed immediately.

Key Points

- Advanced cancer does not mean no treatment
- The focus shifts to control and comfort
- Palliative care improves quality of life
- Pain and symptoms can be managed
- Emotional and family support are essential

Chapter Summary

Advanced cancer requires a compassionate and practical approach. While cure may not be possible, treatment can still control the disease and improve comfort.

Palliative care plays a central role in maintaining quality of life, supported by emotional care and family involvement.

Action Plan

- Discuss treatment goals clearly
- Consider palliative care early
- Report symptoms promptly
- Seek emotional support
- Communicate your preferences
- Focus on comfort and quality of life

Bridge to Next Chapter

While this chapter addresses advanced care, many patients complete treatment and move forward.

In the next chapter, we will discuss life after cancer, including recovery, follow-up, and long-term health.

CHAPTER 17: Life After Cancer: Recovery, Follow-Up, and Moving Forward with Confidence

The End of Treatment Is the Beginning of a New Phase

When cancer treatment ends, many patients expect to feel a sense of closure.

Relief is certainly there. The long journey of treatment has been completed. But along with relief, another feeling often appears quietly.

Uncertainty.

I have heard patients say, "Doctor, treatment is over, but I don't feel completely normal yet."
Others say, "I keep thinking, what if it comes back?"

These feelings are real and very common.

Life after cancer is not simply about returning to the past. It is about moving forward with a new understanding of health and life.

Recovery Takes Time

Your body has gone through a lot.

Treatment may have included surgery, medications, radiation, and emotional stress.

It is natural that recovery takes time.

You may notice:

- Fatigue that improves slowly
- Changes in appetite
- Emotional ups and downs

This is part of the healing process.

Be patient with yourself.

Follow-Up Care: A Critical Part of Your Journey

Even after successful treatment, regular follow-up is essential.

Follow-up care helps to:

- Detect any recurrence early
- Monitor long-term effects of treatment
- Provide reassurance

Follow-up visits may include:

- Physical examination

- Blood tests
- Imaging studies

The schedule depends on your specific situation.

Consistency is important.

Fear of Recurrence: A Natural Feeling

Many patients live with a quiet concern that cancer may return.

This fear is usually stronger in the early months after treatment.

Let me reassure you.

This feeling is normal.

The goal is not to eliminate this fear completely, but to manage it.

Helpful Approaches

- Stay informed, but avoid excessive searching
- Follow your doctor's advice
- Keep regular follow-up appointments
- Focus on daily life rather than constant worry

Over time, this fear usually becomes less intense.

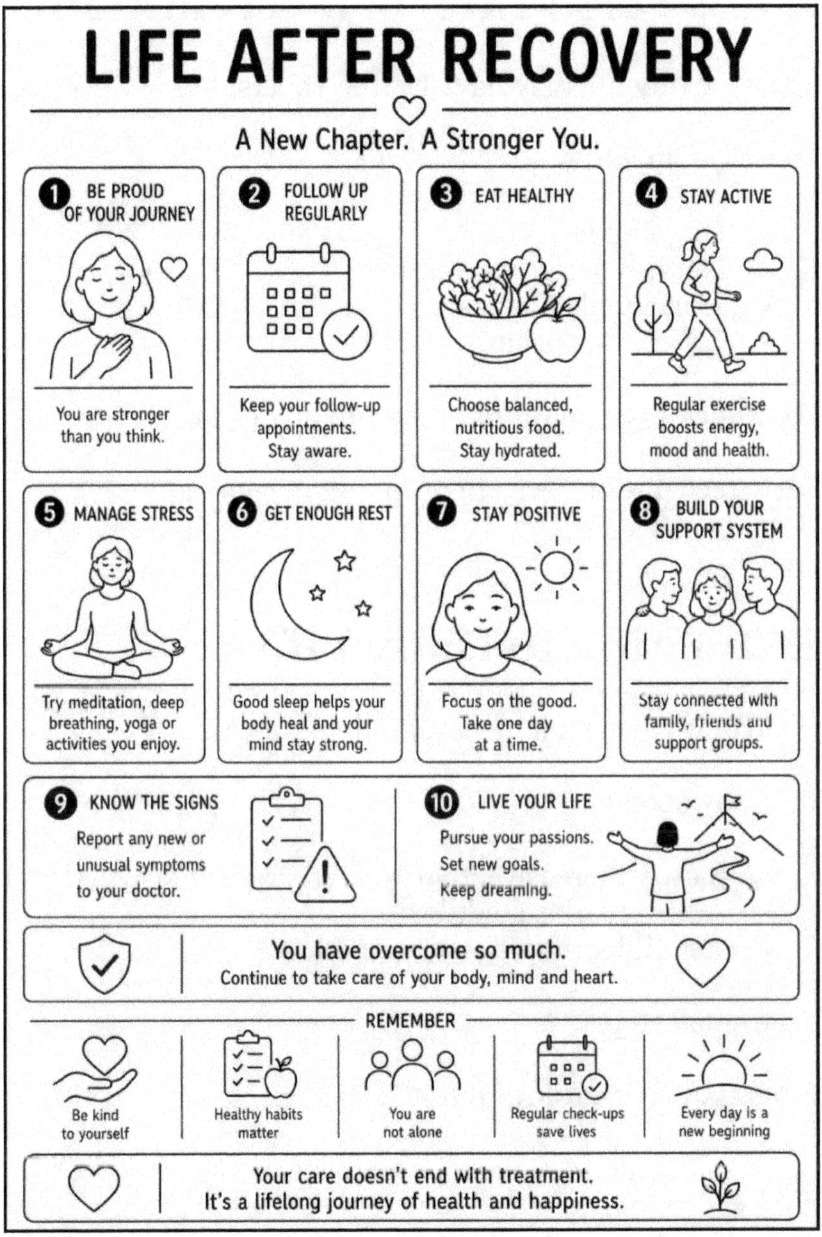
LIFE AFTER RECOVERY
A New Chapter. A Stronger You.
1 BE PROUD OF YOUR JOURNEY
You are stronger than you think.
2 FOLLOW UP REGULARLY
Keep your follow-up appointments. Stay aware.
3 EAT HEALTHY
Choose balanced, nutritious food. Stay hydrated.
4 STAY ACTIVE
Regular exercise boosts energy, mood and health.
5 MANAGE STRESS
Try meditation, deep breathing, yoga or activities you enjoy.
6 GET ENOUGH REST
Good sleep helps your body heal and your mind stay strong.
7 STAY POSITIVE
Focus on the good. Take one day at a time.
8 BUILD YOUR SUPPORT SYSTEM
Stay connected with family, friends and support groups.
9 KNOW THE SIGNS
Report any new or unusual symptoms to your doctor.
10 LIVE YOUR LIFE
Pursue your passions. Set new goals. Keep dreaming.
You have overcome so much.
Continue to take care of your body, mind and heart.
REMEMBER
Be kind to yourself
Healthy habits matter
You are not alone
Regular check-ups save lives
Every day is a new beginning
Your care doesn't end with treatment.
It's a lifelong journey of health and happiness.

Long-Term Effects of Treatment

Some treatments may have lasting effects.

These can include:

- Ongoing fatigue
- Nerve-related symptoms
- Hormonal changes
- Effects on specific organs

Your doctor will monitor these and guide you.

Early recognition helps in proper management.

Returning to Daily Life

Returning to normal life is a gradual process.

You may need to:

- Slowly increase activity
- Adjust work schedules
- Rebuild strength and stamina

Take small steps.

Progress may feel slow, but it is steady.

Reducing the Risk of Recurrence

While recurrence cannot always be prevented, certain steps can help reduce risk.

These include:

- Maintaining a healthy weight
- Eating a balanced diet
- Staying physically active
- Avoiding tobacco
- Limiting alcohol

These are the same principles discussed earlier, now even more important.

Emotional Healing

Recovery is not only physical.

Emotionally, you may experience:

- Anxiety
- Reflection on life priorities
- A deeper awareness of health

Talking about your feelings can help.

Support may come from:

- Family and friends
- Support groups
- Counseling

You do not have to go through this alone.

Supporting Your Family

Your family has been part of your journey.

They may also carry concerns and fears.

Open communication helps:

- Share your progress
- Discuss concerns
- Support each other

Recovery is stronger when shared.

A New Perspective

Many patients tell me that cancer changes how they see life.

They begin to:

- Value health more
- Prioritize relationships
- Focus on what truly matters

This is not just recovery.

It is growth.

A Practical Example

One patient neglects follow-up and returns to unhealthy habits.

Another stays engaged with medical care and maintains a healthy lifestyle.

Over time, their outcomes and confidence may differ significantly.

Doctor's Pearl

Regular follow-up and healthy habits are your strongest protection after treatment.

Myth vs Fact

Myth: Once treatment ends, no further care is needed.
Fact: Follow-up care is essential for long-term health.

Common Mistake to Avoid

Skipping follow-up appointments or ignoring new symptoms.

Red Flag Warning

Any new or persistent symptom after treatment should be evaluated promptly.

Key Points

- Recovery takes time
- Follow-up care is essential
- Fear of recurrence is normal
- Healthy lifestyle reduces risk
- Emotional support is important
- Life after cancer requires adjustment

Chapter Summary

Life after cancer is a phase of recovery, adjustment, and growth. While treatment may be complete, ongoing care remains important.

Regular follow-up, healthy habits, and emotional support help maintain long-term health and confidence.

Action Plan

- Attend all follow-up appointments
- Maintain a healthy lifestyle

- Report new symptoms promptly
- Support your emotional health
- Stay connected with your support system
- Take recovery one step at a time

Bridge to Next Chapter

Even with modern medical knowledge, many myths about cancer still persist.

In the next chapter, we will address common myths and frequently asked questions to help you separate fact from fiction with clarity and confidence.

CHAPTER 18: Cancer Myths and Frequently Asked Questions: Clearing the Confusion

Why Myths About Cancer Still Exist

Even today, many beliefs about cancer are shaped more by fear and past experiences than by current medical knowledge.

People hear stories from friends, relatives, or online sources. Some of these are helpful. Many are incomplete or incorrect.

Over the years, I have seen how these myths can:

- Create unnecessary fear
- Delay proper treatment
- Lead to poor decisions

Clearing these misconceptions is not just about knowledge.

It is about protecting your health.

Myth: Cancer Always Means Death

This is one of the most common fears.

The Truth

Many cancers are treatable, and some are curable, especially when detected early.

Even when cure is not possible, treatment can:

- Control the disease
- Reduce symptoms
- Improve quality of life

Cancer is serious, but it is not always fatal.

Myth: Biopsy Causes Cancer to Spread

This concern is frequently expressed.

The Truth

Biopsy is a safe and essential procedure.

It does not cause cancer to spread in routine medical practice.

Without biopsy, accurate diagnosis is not possible.

Myth: Sugar Directly Feeds Cancer

This idea is widely discussed.

The Truth

All cells in the body use glucose for energy.

Eating sugar does not directly cause cancer growth in a simple way.

However, excessive sugar intake can lead to obesity, which increases cancer risk.

A balanced diet is the key.

Myth: Alternative Treatments Can Cure Cancer

This is a dangerous misconception.

The Truth

There is no reliable scientific evidence that alternative therapies alone can cure cancer.

Some may help with comfort or stress, but they should not replace standard medical treatment.

Delaying proper treatment can worsen outcomes.

Myth: No Symptoms Means No Cancer

The Truth

Many cancers do not produce symptoms in early stages.

That is why screening is important.

Waiting for symptoms may delay diagnosis.

Myth: Cancer Is Always Hereditary

The Truth

Most cancers are not inherited.

Only a small percentage are linked to genetic factors.

Lifestyle and environmental factors play a larger role.

Frequently Asked Questions

Can cancer be cured?

Some cancers can be cured, especially when detected early. Others can be controlled for long periods.

Is treatment always very difficult?

Not necessarily. Many treatments are well tolerated, and side effects can be managed.

Can I continue normal activities during treatment?

In many cases, yes. You may need to adjust based on your energy level.

Do I need a special diet?

No extreme diet is required. A balanced diet is most important.

How do I know what information to trust?

Rely on your doctor and trusted medical sources.

The Role of Accurate Information

Accurate information allows you to:

- Make better decisions
- Avoid unnecessary fear
- Seek timely care

In contrast, misinformation can lead to delay and confusion.

Hope with Realism

It is important to remain balanced.

Not every cancer can be cured.

But progress in medicine is real.

New treatments continue to improve outcomes and quality of life.

Hope should be based on facts, not false promises.

A Practical Example

One patient relies on myths and delays treatment.

Another seeks reliable information and follows medical advice.

The second patient is more likely to receive timely and effective care.

Doctor's Pearl

Accurate information is as important as treatment.

Common Mistake to Avoid

Believing unverified claims and delaying proper care.

Red Flag Warning

Be cautious of any claim that promises a guaranteed cure without scientific evidence.

Key Points

- Many cancer myths are incorrect
- Cancer does not always mean death
- Biopsy is safe
- No single food or remedy cures cancer

- Early detection and proper treatment matter
- Reliable information is essential

Chapter Summary

Cancer myths can create fear and lead to poor decisions. Understanding the facts allows you to approach cancer with clarity and confidence.

Reliable, evidence-based information is essential for making the right choices.

Action Plan

- Rely on trusted medical advice
- Avoid unverified claims
- Discuss doubts with your doctor
- Stay informed with reliable sources
- Focus on evidence-based care

Bridge to Final Chapter

You have now gained a clear understanding of cancer, from its causes and prevention to diagnosis and treatment.

In the final chapter, we will bring everything together and focus on how you can take control of your health with confidence.

CHAPTER 19: From Fear to Control: Taking Charge of Your Health

Looking Back: From Uncertainty to Understanding

If you have read this far, you have already taken a very important step.

You have chosen to understand.

We began with fear, which is natural when facing a word like cancer. Step by step, we moved through what cancer is, why it happens, how it can be prevented, how it is detected, and how it is treated.

We discussed difficult situations as well as hopeful ones.

Now, you are no longer looking at cancer as an unknown.

You are looking at it with clarity.

The Most Important Truth: You Are Not Helpless

One of the greatest burdens cancer brings is the feeling of losing control.

But the truth is different.

You are not helpless.

There are meaningful actions you can take:

- You can reduce your risk
- You can recognize early warning signs
- You can follow screening recommendations
- You can seek timely medical care
- You can make informed decisions

These actions may seem simple, but they are powerful.

The Power of Early Action

If there is one message that stands above the rest, it is this:

Early action makes a difference.

Many cancers:

- Develop slowly
- Can be detected early
- Can be treated effectively when found early

Delays often lead to more complex situations.

Timely attention leads to better outcomes.

Health Is Built Over Time

Good health is not created in a single day.

It is built through daily habits.

Simple steps make a difference:

- Eating a balanced diet
- Staying physically active
- Avoiding tobacco
- Limiting alcohol
- Maintaining a healthy weight

These are not temporary measures.

They are long-term commitments.

Working with Your Doctor

Your doctor is your partner in health.

Good communication improves care.

- Ask questions
- Share concerns
- Understand your options
- Follow medical advice

When you are involved, your care becomes stronger.

Staying Informed Without Being Overwhelmed

Information today is everywhere.

But not all information is reliable.

Choose your sources carefully.

Focus on:

- Your doctor's guidance
- Trusted medical organizations

Avoid confusion by limiting exposure to unreliable or conflicting information.

Your Role in Your Family's Health

Your actions do not affect only you.

They influence those around you.

By taking care of your health, you:

- Set an example
- Encourage awareness
- Support your family

Health awareness often spreads from one person to many.

Living with Awareness, Not Fear

Fear has a role. It can make us alert.

But it should not control our lives.

Awareness is different.

Awareness allows you to:

- Notice changes
- Take timely action
- Make informed choices

You do not need to live in constant worry.

You need to stay aware.

A Practical Example

Two individuals have similar risks.

One ignores symptoms and avoids screening.

The other stays aware and takes timely action.

The difference in outcomes often comes from awareness and action.

Doctor's Pearl

Awareness, early action, and healthy habits are your strongest protection.

Myth vs Fact

Myth: Nothing can be done to prevent cancer.
Fact: Many cancers can be prevented or detected early.

Common Mistake to Avoid

Ignoring health until symptoms become serious.

Red Flag Warning

Do not delay medical evaluation for persistent or unexplained symptoms.

Key Points

- You are not helpless
- Early detection improves outcomes
- Healthy habits reduce risk
- Communication with your doctor is essential
- Awareness leads to better decisions

Chapter Summary

Cancer is a serious condition, but understanding it gives you the ability to take meaningful control of your health. Prevention, awareness, early detection, and informed decisions are the foundation of effective care.

This book has been written to guide you toward clarity, confidence, and practical action.

Final Action Plan

- Maintain a healthy lifestyle
- Avoid tobacco
- Stay physically active
- Follow recommended screening
- Pay attention to warning signs
- Seek medical advice promptly
- Stay informed through reliable sources
- Encourage your family to stay healthy

A Final Thought

Cancer is a word that brings fear.

But fear should not guide your life.

Understanding should.

With knowledge, awareness, and timely action, you can face this challenge with confidence.

Take care of your health.

Stay aware.

And remember, you have more control than you think.

APPENDIX 1: SIMPLE CANCER SCREENING GUIDE (BY AGE AND RISK)

Why This Appendix Matters

One of the most practical things you can take away from this book is knowing **when to get screened**.

Screening saves lives. It helps detect cancer early, sometimes even before symptoms appear.

This guide is simple, practical, and based on widely accepted medical recommendations. Individual needs may vary, so always confirm with your doctor.

General Principles to Remember

- Screening is for people without symptoms
- Recommendations depend on age, gender, and risk factors
- Family history may require earlier or more frequent screening
- Consistency is more important than perfection

Screening for Adults (General Population)

Age 20–39

- **Cervical cancer (women)**
  Pap test starting at age 21, every 3 years
- **Breast awareness (women)**
  Be familiar with your breast and report any changes
- **General health check-ups**
  Periodic evaluation based on individual risk

Age 40–49

- **Breast cancer (women)**
  Mammography may begin based on individual risk
- **Cervical cancer (women)**
  Continue Pap test or combined Pap + HPV testing
- **Colon cancer**
  Begin screening earlier if family history exists

Age 50–74

- **Breast cancer (women)**
  Mammography every 1–2 years
- **Colon cancer (men and women)**
  - Colonoscopy every 10 years, or
  - Stool-based tests as recommended
- **Cervical cancer (women)**
  Continue screening as advised
- **Prostate cancer (men)**
  PSA testing after discussion with your doctor

Age 55–80 (High-Risk Individuals)

- **Lung cancer screening**
  Annual low-dose CT scan for long-term smokers

When Screening May Be Needed Earlier

You may need earlier or more frequent screening if you have:

- Strong family history of cancer
- Genetic risk factors
- Long-term tobacco use
- Certain chronic infections

Always discuss your personal risk with your doctor.

When to Stop Screening

Screening decisions later in life depend on:

- Overall health
- Life expectancy
- Previous screening results

These decisions should be individualized.

Doctor's Pearl

Screening is most effective when done regularly and at the right time.

Key Points

- Screening detects cancer early
- It is done even when you feel well
- Recommendations vary by age and risk
- Consistency is essential

APPENDIX 2: 30-DAY CANCER PREVENTION AND HEALTH PLAN

Why This Plan Matters

Many people want to improve their health but are unsure where to start.

This simple 30-day plan provides a structured approach.

It is not extreme. It is practical and sustainable.

WEEK 1: Building Awareness

- Observe your daily habits
- Identify unhealthy patterns
- Start reducing processed foods
- Begin light physical activity (10–15 minutes daily)

WEEK 2: Making Small Changes

- Increase fruits and vegetables
- Drink more water
- Walk 20–30 minutes daily

- Reduce alcohol intake

WEEK 3: Strengthening Habits

- Maintain regular meal timing
- Add simple strength exercises
- Improve sleep routine
- Practice stress reduction techniques

WEEK 4: Creating Consistency

- Continue all healthy habits
- Review your progress
- Adjust what is not working
- Set long-term goals

Doctor's Pearl

Small, consistent changes over time create lasting health benefits.

Key Points

- Start small
- Stay consistent

- Avoid extreme changes
- Focus on long-term habits

APPENDIX 3: QUESTIONS TO ASK YOUR DOCTOR

Why Asking Questions Matters

Clear communication improves care.

Patients who ask questions understand their condition better and make more confident decisions.

Questions After Diagnosis

- What type of cancer do I have?
- What stage is it?
- Has it spread?
- What is the goal of treatment?

Questions About Treatment

- What are my treatment options?
- What are the benefits and risks?
- What side effects should I expect?
- How will treatment affect my daily life?

Questions About Follow-Up

- How often do I need check-ups?
- What symptoms should I watch for?
- How can I reduce the risk of recurrence?

Doctor's Pearl

There are no wrong questions when it comes to your health.

Key Points

- Ask clear questions
- Take notes
- Bring support to appointments
- Stay involved in your care

FINAL NOTE (END OF BOOK)

This book was written to simplify a complex subject.

Cancer is serious, but understanding it changes how you respond to it.

When you understand:

- You act earlier
- You decide better
- You live with more confidence

That is the true purpose of this book.

Thank You and Please Review the Book

Thank you for taking the time to read this book. I sincerely hope it has helped you understand your health a little more clearly and has given you practical, everyday steps you can follow with confidence. If you found this book helpful, **I would truly appreciate it if you could leave a brief and honest review.** Even a few lines sharing your experience can make a meaningful difference. Your feedback helps other readers find reliable, trustworthy health information and supports them in making better decisions for themselves and their families.

Warm regards,

Dr Prabhat Das

Continue your Healthcare Journey with these Books

Good health is a journey, not a single step. It is not achieved in one day or with one book. That is why I created the "Better Health with Dr Das Series", with each book addressing a different common condition. If you would like easy, practical guidance on other everyday health concerns, you may wish to explore the rest of books in this series.

Books in this series:

- Better Health starts Here: A Doctor's Guide to Staying Healthy After 40
- A Doctor's Easy Guide to Understanding & Managing OBESITY
- Doctor, What DIET Is Best for Me?
- Doctor, Why Can't I Lose Weight? A Doctor's Guide to Safe & Sustainable Weight Loss)
- A Doctor's Easy Guide to GLP-1 for Obesity
- A Doctor's Easy Guide to Understanding & Managing HIGH BLOOD PRESSURE
- A Doctor's Guide to Living Well With DIABETES
- A Doctor's Guide to Understanding & Managing THYROID DISEASES
- A Doctor's Guide to Understanding & Managing HIGH CHOLESTEROL
- A Doctor's Practical Guide to HEART HEALTH After 40: How to Protect Your Heart & Live Longer
- A Doctor's Guide to Healing & Reversing FATTY LIVER DISEASE: Simple, Natural & Science-Based Steps to Reduce Liver Fat and Prevent Complications

- Control Your ACID REFLUX, HEARTBURN & GERD: A Doctor's Practical Guide that Works
- Live Comfortably with IRRITABLE BOWEL SYNDROME: A Doctor's Practical Guide to Understanding & Managing IBS
- A Doctor's Practical Guide to Understanding & Managing GALLBLADDER STONES & OTHER PROBLEMS
- Take Control of COPD: A Doctor's Practical Guide to Better Breathing
- Living Better with ASTHMA: A Doctor's Practical Guide to Asthma Control
- SLEEP APNEA, INSOMNIA & OTHER SLEEP DISORDERS: A Doctor's Practical Guide to Better Sleep & Better Health
- Protect Your KIDNEYS: A Doctor's Practical Guide to Kidney Health & Prevention
- PROSTATE HEALTH: A Doctor's Practical Guide to Early Detection & Care
- ARTHRITIS: A Doctor's Practical Guide to Pain Control & Mobility
- STROKE: A Doctor's Practical Guide to Prevention & Early detection
- HEART ATTACK: A Doctor's Practical Guide to Prevention & Early detection
- CANCER: A Doctor's Practical Guide to Prevention & Early detection
- BACK PAIN: A Doctor's Practical Guide to Fixing Step by Step
- COMMON SKIN & HAIR PROBLEMS: A Doctor's Practical Guide to Skin & Hair Care
- DEMENTIA & MEMORY LOSS: A Doctor's Practical Guide to Prevention & Management
- Doctor, Why Am I TIRED All the Time? Fixing Fatigue & Getting Your Energy Back

www.ingramcontent.com/pod-product-compliance
Lightning Source LLC
LaVergne TN
LVHW020854300926
849194LV00002B/13